OPTIMUM
NUTRITION
for your
Child's Mind

OPTIMUM NUTRITION
for your Child's Mind

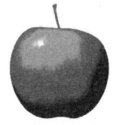

Maximise your child's potential

PATRICK HOLFORD

& DEBORAH COLSON

PIATKUS

Visit the Piatkus website!

Piatkus publishes a wide range of best-selling fiction and non-fiction, including books on health, mind, body & spirit, sex, self-help, cookery, biography and the paranormal.

If you want to:
- read descriptions of our popular titles
- buy our books over the Internet
- take advantage of our special offers
- enter our monthly competition
- learn more about your favourite Piatkus authors

VISIT OUR WEBSITE AT: www.piatkus.co.uk

Copyright © 2006 by Patrick Holford and Deborah Colson

First published in Great Britain in 2006 by
Piatkus Books Ltd
5 Windmill Street, London W1T 2JA
email: info@piatkus.co.uk

Reprinted 2006

The moral right of the author has been asserted

A catalogue record for this book is available from the British Library

ISBN 0 7499 2685 6

Edited by Barbara Kiser
Text design by Briony Chappell

This book has been printed on paper manufactured with respect for the environment using wood from managed sustainable resources

Typeset in Great Britain by Phoenix Photosetting, Chatham, Kent
Printed and bound in Great Britain by William Clowes Ltd, Beccles, Suffolk

CONTENTS

Acknowledgements   viii
Guide to Abbreviations, Measures and References   ix
References and Further Sources of Information   x
Introduction   1

PART 1 – FOOD FOR THE BRAIN   **9**
1   How Food Builds the Brain   11
2   No Sugar, Thanks – I'm Sweet Enough Already   20
3   Smart Fats – The Mind's Construction Crew   39
4   Phospholipids – Go to School on an Egg   55
5   Protein – The Architect of Mind and Mood   60
6   Why Vitamins and Minerals Make Your Child Brainy   67
7   Don't Let Your Child be a Heavy Metal Kid   78
8   Keeping Your Child Chemical Free   85
9   Protecting Your Child from Brain Allergies   93

PART 2 – GIVE YOUR CHILD A HEAD START   **101**
10   Testing, Testing   103
11   Thinking Faster, Boosting IQ   107
12   Developing Concentration and a Sharp Memory   117
13   Revving Up Reading and Writing   127
14   Enhancing Mood and Behaviour   135

PART 3 – SOLVING PROBLEMS   **147**
15   Dyslexia and Dyspraxia – What Works   149
16   Drug-Free Solutions for ADHD   155

17 Moving Off the Autistic Spectrum   170
18 Answers for Aggression   193
19 Overcoming Eating Disorders   199
20 Curing Sleeping Problems   209

PART 4 – FOOD FOR THOUGHT   **217**
21 Getting off to a Good Start   219
22 Preventing Food Fads and Fussiness   228
23 Guerrilla Tactics in the Supermarket   233
24 Top Tips in the Kitchen   238
25 Making Healthy Meals at School Cool   245
26 Supplements for Superkids   249
27 Join the Food for the Brain Campaign   254

REFERENCES AND RESOURCES   **257**
References   257
Recommended Reading   273
Resources   274
Product and Supplement Directory   280
Index   286

ACKNOWLEDGEMENTS

We'd like to thank the many scientists, such as Dr Alex Richardson, Bernard Gesch and Professor Michael Crawford, who have tirelessly put the role of optimum nutrition for children's brain development on the map, often funding their own research. Enormous thanks go to Susannah Lawson, co-author of *Optimum Nutrition Before During and After Pregnancy*, for her many contributions. Also to Jo and Barbara, our wonderful, painstaking editors at Piatkus. But, most of all we'd like to thank the many children and their parents who we've worked with at the Brain Bio Centre: it is they who have taught us the most.

GUIDE TO ABBREVIATIONS, MEASURES AND REFERENCES

Abbreviations and measures

1 gram (g) = 1,000 milligrams (mg) = 1,000,000 micrograms (mcg, also written μg).

All vitamins are measured in milligrams or micrograms. Vitamins A, D and E used to be measured in International Units (ius), a measurement designed to standardise the various forms of these vitamins that have different potencies.

6mcg of beta-carotene, the vegetable precursor of vitamin A, is, on average, converted into 1mcg of retinol, the animal form of vitamin A. So, 6mcg of betacarotene is called 1mcgRE (RE stands for retinol equivalent). Throughout this book beta-carotene is referred to in mcgRE.

1mcg of retinol (mcgRE) = 3.3ius of vitamin A
1mcgRE of beta-carotene = 6mcg of beta-carotene
100ius of vitamin D = 2.5mcg
100ius of vitamin E = 67mg
1 pound (lb) = 16 ounces (oz)   2.2lb = 1 kilogram (kg)
1 pint = 0.6 litres 1.76 pints = 1 litre
In this book calories means kilocalories (kcals)

REFERENCES AND FURTHER SOURCES OF INFORMATION

Hundreds of references from respected scientific literature have been used in the writing of this book. Details of specific studies referred to are listed on pages 257–272. Other supporting research for statements made is available from the library at the Institute for Optimum Nutrition (ION) (see page 274). ION also offers information services, including literature search and library search facilities, for those readers who want to access scientific literature on specific subjects. On page 273 you will find a list of the best books to read to enable you to dig deeper into the topics covered. You will also find many of the topics touched on in this book covered in detail in Patrick's feature articles, available at www.patrickholford.com If you want to stay up to date with all that is new and exciting in this field we recommend you subscribe to Patrick's *100% Health* newsletter, details of which are on the website.

INTRODUCTION

All parents have an instinct to help their children be all they can. We want our children to be happy, intelligent and resourceful, with the full range of life skills they'll need to live productively and well. That is, in essence, what childhood is all about.

We teach our children how to eat, how to walk and talk, how to get the most out of what they're learning at school. We give them as much love and attention as we can to enable them to develop physically, mentally and emotionally. We read books about parenting, we try not to make the same mistakes our parents made, we struggle over choosing the right school to support our child through the process of becoming an adult and finding their way in the world.

But through all of this, do we really take into account the fact that every step a child takes – whether it's their first toddle on the kitchen floor, or their sudden plunge into emotions and relationships as teenagers – depends on how well their brain is working? And that, in turn, depends in large part on how well their brain is nourished?

From plate to brain

This is a 'how to' book. Whether your child is one year old or 15, you want to know what you can do to help them be all they can be – and you'll discover how in these pages. Armed with more than 20 years' experience of working with children, we are going to show you, step by step, what optimum nutrition for your child's mind really means.

At long last, governments and schools are cottoning on to children's need for a truly well-balanced diet rather than the junk-food afterthought they've had to put up with. Society is waking up to the fact that schools have a moral responsibility to give children good food, aware – through media exposés such as Jamie Oliver's – that the quality of school dinners has long been too low a priority.

Why has this grim state of affairs persisted so long? Simply because food has been misperceived as fuel – so that, if a child is full after a meal and isn't showing obvious signs of malnourishment, it's seen as 'good enough'.

But the true picture lies in how you read the signs in a child's behaviour or appearance. Take intelligence. Somehow embedded in our culture is the false idea that this is inherited, and there's nothing you can do about it. I (Patrick) trained as a psychologist and I've always had a keen interest in our intellectual development. As the brain is essentially made from the food we eat, I was already wondering back in the 1980s whether giving children extra vitamins and minerals could boost their intelligence.

Working with secondary school head Gwillym Roberts and Professor David Benton from the University of Wales in Swansea, we proved that you can dramatically boost a child's IQ just by making changes in their nutrition – an experiment showcased in a 1988 BBC documentary. In the study, we measured the IQ scores of 90 schoolchildren and then gave 30 of them a high-dose multivitamin, 30 a dummy pill and 30 nothing. After eight months we re-evaluated their IQ. Only those children on the vitamins had a staggering increase in their IQs of over ten points![1]

This study, the first of its kind anywhere in the world, raised a new question: How can you keep your child's mind optimally nourished?

Nutrition in mind

If there is a difference between the learning and behaviour of kids who eat junk food with abandon and those who are following the so-called 'well-balanced diet', what is that difference, why is there a difference and what exactly should you, as a parent, be feeding your child? These are the questions we've lived and breathed for the past 20 years.

As you'll see in this book, study after study shows that you can increase intelligence, attention span, concentration, problem-solving ability, emotional response, mood, physical coordination – all the facets of intelligence – simply by changing what goes into and onto their bowls, plates and lunchboxes.

While the practical advice we'll be giving you is based on solid scientific research, we feel even more confident about our conclusions because we have worked with hundreds of children over the past two decades. Some of them were disabled, some coping with serious behavioural problems – yet all were transformed once their own unique optimum nutrition needs were discovered, and fulfilled.

Every day at the London clinic of the Brain Bio Centre, at the Institute for Optimum Nutrition founded by Patrick in 1984, we see children who are struggling to learn, develop and adapt. I (Deborah) am a nutritional therapist specialising in children's development. My job is not only to find out what's wrong – be it a food allergy, a chemical sensitivity or a nutrient deficiency – but also to show parents how to make good food that children like, weaning them off sugar and expanding the range of healthy foods on the daily menu.

As well as working one-to-one with kids and parents at the

Brain Bio Centre, we've tested our theories in primary schools, secondary schools and special schools for disadvantaged children. ITV's *This Morning* programme, for example, gave us one week to improve the learning of a class of seven- to eight-year-olds. Later on you'll read the story of Reece, a 'hyperactive' child in this class whose reading level went up a year in one month on the diet.

Tonight with Trevor McDonald gave us three badly behaved boys – one of whom was Liam (see page 144) – all of whom had been kicked out of mainstream schools, and asked us to get them back on track in a month. You'll find out what happened to these boys, too, along with the supplements we've recommended for all these kids, and how a simple test can reveal whether your child's brain is working at its best.

Much of our work has been with children and young adults diagnosed with ADHD, autism, Asperger's, depression, even psychosis. The usual route for children with these conditions is prescription drugs, or specialised psychological support. We believe that optimum nutrition is a vital aspect of helping these children discover, or recover, their full potential. Consider these studies:

- Bernard Gesch, director of the charity Natural Justice, gave some of Britain's worst young offenders supplements of vitamins, minerals and essential fats, or placebos, and demonstrated a dramatic 35 per cent decrease in aggressive acts, in two weeks, only in those taking the supplements.[2]

- Dr Alexandra Richardson of the University of Oxford conducted a randomised controlled trial with 117 children aged 5 to 12 who had coordination problems. The children who received supplements of omega-3 and omega-6 fatty acids showed significant improvements in reading, spelling and behaviour over three months compared to those who didn't receive the supplements.[3]

- Researchers from Örebro University in Sweden compared the school grades in ten core subjects with homocysteine levels in a group of 692 school children aged 9 to 15. (Homocysteine is an indicator of B vitamin deficiency.) Higher homocysteine levels were strongly associated with lower grades.[4]

- Researchers at the Institute of Child Health in London placed 78 hyperactive children on a 'few foods' diet, which eliminates both chemical additives and common food allergens. The behaviour of 59 of the children, or 76 per cent, improved during this open trial. To check whether the foods would affect the children's behaviour if no one knew whether they were eating them or not, the researchers managed to disguise the foods and additives that provoked reactions in 19 of the children. When these children were given the disguised offending foods, their behaviour ratings and performance in psychological testing both worsened.[5]

- Dr Bernard Rimland from California compared 1,591 hyperactive children treated with drugs to 191 hyperactive children given nutritional supplements. The nutritional approach was 18 times more effective at reducing hyperactivity.[6] Yet, despite this, drug prescriptions for children nearly double every year.

If simple changes in nutrition can have such profound effects on the young people in these studies, isn't it likely that optimum nutrition can help your child reach their full potential? That means every child – not just children with conditions such as autism, hyperactivity or behavioural problems. Optimum nutrition can sharpen up your child's mind and mood even if you feel they are doing 'all right'.

As you follow the guidelines in this book, you will notice gradual improvements in their ability to learn and behave. You really can change how your child thinks, feels and behaves by changing what goes into their mouth, and we're going to show you how.

By doing so, you'll be in the vanguard of teachers, health professionals and other concerned parents who are leading a revolution in food awareness. Although governments are waking up to the implications of all the new research, they have not yet accepted across the board just how profoundly nutrition can influence learning and behaviour. In the UK, for example, over £240 million was spent last year on psychological interventions in school for children with learning or behavioural problems. And how much was spent on the kind of highly effective nutritional intervention we describe in this book? Precisely nothing.

The time is ripe for change, and you can help make it happen.

How to use this book

In Part 1, 'Food for the Brain', you'll discover the five essential brain foods, an optimum intake of which is essential for maximising your child's potential. There are also five 'anti-nutrients' that can disrupt and damage the brain and are best avoided. This part shows you what to feed your child, and what to avoid.

In Part 2, 'Give Your Child a Head Start', you'll discover the foods and supplements that are proven to boost IQ, improve mood and behaviour, sharpen memory and concentration and improve reading and writing. In this part of the book, you will discover how to maximise your child's potential for better school performance, happiness and personal fulfilment.

In Part 3, 'Solving Problems', we give you nutritional solutions for children with conditions such as autism, hyperactivity and aggression to help you maximise their potential for mental and emotional health.

In Part 4, 'Food for Thought', we'll show you how to put this into action, explaining what to do to feed your child properly, from infancy to teenage years. You'll find plenty of shopping tips, meal ideas and practical ways of keeping your child's diet on track, as well as how to choose the right supplements.

The biggest gift we can give our children is getting them off to the best start in life, socially and academically. A huge part of that is to make available to them the best nutrition, to help them feel alert, energetic, happy and unstressed, with a clear mind and a focused intelligence. This book is written with that goal in mind.

Wishing you and your children the best of health,

Patrick Holford and Deborah Colson

PART 1

Food for the Brain

Food directly affects how your child thinks and feels because their brains (and yours) are made of it. There are five essential brain foods – slow-release carbohydrates, essential fats, phospholipids, amino acids, and vitamins and minerals. An optimum intake of these is essential for maximising your child's potential. Then there are the five 'anti-nutrients', substances that can disrupt and damage the brain – refined sugar, damaged fats, certain chemical food additives, toxic minerals and food allergens. These are best avoided. In this part of the book you'll find out what, and what not, to feed your child.

CHAPTER 1

How Food Builds the Brain

One of the most limiting concepts in the human sciences is the idea that mind and body are separate. Try asking an anatomist, a psychologist and a biochemist where the mind begins and the body ends. It is a stupid question, and yet that is exactly what modern science has done by separating psychology from medicine. Few psychologists know much about brain chemistry and the importance of nutrition, and few doctors know enough about the psychological or nutritional factors that affect a child's development.

But it's not just the scientists who live by this false dichotomy. It's all of us. It's undoubtedly second nature to you to help your child grow physically strong and healthy. But when they're having difficulty concentrating, behaving badly or struggling to read, does the thought that they might be poorly nourished cross your mind? If it doesn't, it's vital to know that all these attributes and behaviours are governed by a network of interconnecting brain cells, each of which depends profoundly on what your child puts into his or her mouth.

Many of our children are struggling to keep up. They're living with constant tiredness, difficulty in concentrating, erratic behaviour, anxiety, stress, depression and sleeping problems. Too many children are suffering from mental health problems ranging from attention deficit disorder to autism, hyperactivity and dyslexia; or they're simply not achieving their full potential in school and at home because the way they feel makes it difficult to focus and learn. In fact, the world over there's been a massive rise in the incidence of mental health problems, especially among young people.[7]

By understanding how your child's brain works, you can eradicate these problems and smooth your child's path through their crucial developing years. It will become more than clear why giving a child certain nutrients every day, ideally from conception, can have a profound effect on how they think and feel – and thus, how they behave in the here and now, and how they develop over time.

Brains – what make us human

Our story starts not at birth, but at conception and all the way through pregnancy. Studies of the time we spend in the womb are showing us that human growth and development – unlike that of, say, a rhinoceros – centre largely on the development of the brain. Brains, not brawn, are what make us human.

Take a look at the diagram opposite. A human baby's brain is more than 300 times larger, compared to its body size, than that of a rhinoceros. Size matters – but that's not all. During development in the womb, half of all the nutrition the foetus receives from its mother is directly channelled into feeding brain growth.

This is quite a task. Although a mere 450g (1lb) in weight at birth, your child's brain consumes, and needs, a vast quantity of nutrients, including protein, carbohydrate, vitamins, minerals and essential fats. Fats are a big one here, as the brain is literally made out of it. In fact, if you drained all the water out of a brain, a whopping 60 per cent of it would be fat.

Four specific kinds of fat (known as AA, DHA, EPA and DGLA – more on these later) make up 20 per cent of the brain. So deficiencies of these at any time, but especially during foetal or early development, can have huge repercussions on intelligence and behaviour.

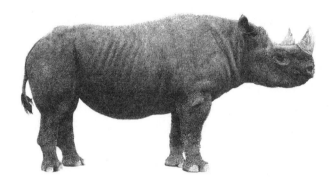

A rhinoceros weighs 1 ton but has a tiny 35g brain, which is 0.035% of its total body weight

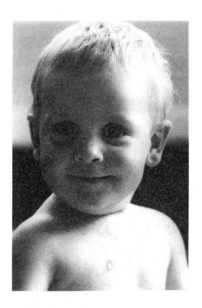

A newborn baby weighs about 4kg and has a 450g brain, which is 11% of its total body weight

So vital are these fats to the growing foetus that it will literally rob its mother's brain to make its own. It's a case of 'Mummy, I shrunk your brain': if a pregnant woman's diet is deficient in the essential fats, her brain will actually get smaller!

At every stage of brain development, achieving optimum nutrition is essential to guarantee that your child achieves his or her full potential. At birth, the level of essential fats in the umbilical cord of a newborn infant correlates with the speed of their thinking at age eight. By the age of eight, the blood level of homocysteine, which is the best indicator of a child's B vitamin status, will correlate with their school grades.[8] If a teenager's daily intake of zinc is just twice the level of the recommended daily allowance (RDA), this can improve attention and concentration to an astonishing degree.[9] And at any age, the intake of anti-nutrients like sugar and damaged fats has proven harmful effects on both learning and behaviour.

If you find these facts hard to believe, you may not be aware how flexible and open to change the human brain is. Let's look at it for a moment to fathom why this is.

Joined-up thinking

As it grows, a foetus builds thousands of brain cells, called neurons, every minute. By the age of two, a child's brain has approximately 100 billion of them. That's a lot – approximately the same number of neurons as there are trees in the Amazon! And just like the interlocking branches of those billions of rainforest trees, the neurons are connected up. So what we call the brain is essentially a network of these specialised nerve cells, all linked up to other neurons.

While the number of neurons doesn't increase in children beyond the age of two, the number of connections made between neurons does, very dramatically. When a baby is born, every neuron in the cerebral cortex – the 'grey matter' and

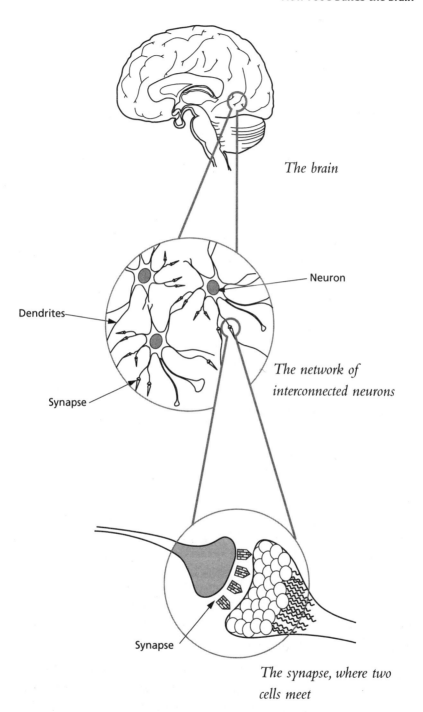

The brain

Neuron

Dendrites

Synapse

The network of interconnected neurons

Synapse

The synapse, where two cells meet

outermost layer of the brain – can connect with about 2,500 other neurons. By the time that child is two or three years old, that number has swollen to 15,000.

These connections are vital to memory, cognition and learning because they're the conduits along which the electrical impulses of our thoughts travel. And children, those master learners, are hard-wiring these connections every minute.

When learning language, for instance, young children will keep repeating words to hard-wire the image they are seeing with the sound they are making, reinforced by your positive feedback. Every thought they think is represented by a 'ripple' of activity across the network of neurons. With repeated thoughts and actions, be it speech or movement, the neuronal pathways are reinforced. Meanwhile, other, redundant connections will get dismantled. Unlike other organs in the body, the brain is always restructuring itself.

Let's take a closer look at the connections between neurons. These are called dendrites, and where one dendrite meets another, there's a gap, like the 'spark' gap in a spark plug. This gap is called a synapse, and it's across it that messages are sent from one neuron to another.

The message is sent from a sending station and received in a receiving station, called a receptor. These sending and receiving stations are built out of essential fats, found in fish and seeds; phospholipids, present in eggs and organ meats; and amino acids, the raw material of protein.

The message itself, known as a neurotransmitter, is in most cases made out of amino acids. Different amino acids make different neurotransmitters. For example, the neurotransmitter serotonin, which keeps you happy, is made from the amino acid tryptophan. Adrenalin and dopamine, which keep you motivated, are made from phenylalanine.

Turning an amino acid into a neurotransmitter is no simple

job. Enzymes in the brain that depend on vitamins, minerals and special amino acids accomplish this task. These vitamins and minerals also control the steady supply of fuel – blood sugar or glucose – that powers each neuron.

From all this, you can see how the food your children eat does more than build their bodies. It's building the very structure of their brains, from the neurons themselves to the messages that shoot from one to another. So food governs how your child thinks and feels to a massive degree.

The basic structure of your child's brain is laid down by

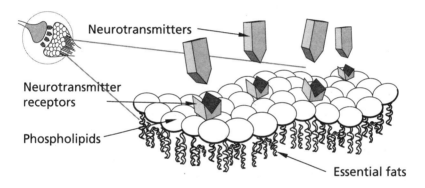

Close-up of a receptor

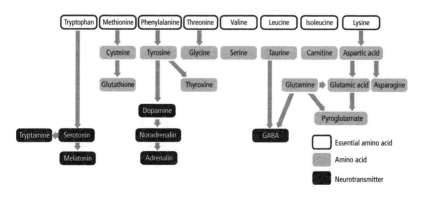

Neurotransmitters are made from amino acids

genetics. But what you feed them, along with what they learn, helps develop that structure, and through that their intelligence and ability to learn, adapt and have a happy and fulfilling life. While you can't change genes, you can change your child's nutrition and learning resources. That's why your biggest task, as a parent, is ensuring optimum nutrition while stimulating your child's inbuilt capacity for learning.

In the context of your child's brain, optimum nutrition is all about choosing five essential foods, and avoiding others. Let's look at them now.

What goes on – or off – the plate

Optimum nutrition means achieving the right intake of the **five essential brain foods**:

- **Balanced blood sugar** – the brain's superfuel

- **Essential fats** – why a 'fathead' is a smart head

- **Phospholipids** – memory molecules that give 'oomph' to the brain

- **Amino acids** – the brain's messengers

- **Vitamins and minerals** – the intelligent nutrients that keep the brain in tune.

But this isn't the whole story. You will also need to **avoid anti-nutrients** – substances that damage the brain:

- **Refined sugar** – carbohydrates robbed of essential nutrients

- **Damaged fats** – from fried food to hydrogenated fats

- **Chemical food additives** – colourings, flavourings and preservatives

- **Toxic minerals** – from copper to mercury

- **Food allergens** – common foods your child might be allergic to.

In the chapters that follow we'll explain how to discover which foods or chemicals your child is particularly sensitive to and would do best to avoid. And the next five chapters explain in detail what the five essential brain foods are, and how to give your child the optimal amount. These chapters explain the basics of optimum nutrition for your child's mind.

CHAPTER 2

No Sugar, Thanks – I'm Sweet Enough Already

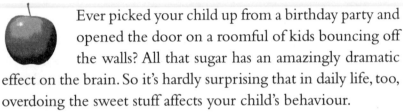 Ever picked your child up from a birthday party and opened the door on a roomful of kids bouncing off the walls? All that sugar has an amazingly dramatic effect on the brain. So it's hardly surprising that in daily life, too, overdoing the sweet stuff affects your child's behaviour.

Yet nothing is more important for your child's brain than sugar – blood sugar, or glucose, that is. It's the brain's main fuel, so without an adequate supply we can't think clearly. We get it from the sugars and starches – in other words, the carbohydrates – in the foods we eat. The trick lies in keeping that supply even.

Too much, and you get the wall-bouncing effect. Too little, and your child could experience symptoms like fatigue, irritability, dizziness, insomnia, aggression, anxiety, sweating (especially at night), poor concentration, excessive thirst, depression, crying spells or blurred vision. So for your child to be able to think with clarity and behave rationally, it's vital that their glucose supply stays steady and even.

John is a case in point. Four-year-old John's parents brought him to see us at the Brain Bio Centre because they were concerned about his severe speech and language delay and his inability to concentrate. We screened him for various biochemical imbalances and analysed his diet. John's diet, while fairly typical for a four-year-old and not especially unhealthy, contained a lot of hidden sugar. We recommended that his parents reduce all sources of sugar as much as possible, including high-GL (glycemic load) fruits such as bananas. Within a few weeks, according to his parents, child minder and teachers, John was a different child. His scribblings had transformed into drawings accompanied by a verbal explanation. He slept better at night and no longer needed to nap during the day. He was much calmer, had improved comprehension and began attempting jigsaw puzzles. John's granddad inadvertently illustrated how sensitive John is to sugar when one day during this period he gave John half a banana, thinking it was allowed on the 'diet'. The effect was incredible. 'He went completely beserk,' recalls John's mum. He ran from one end of the house to the other for an hour until the effect of the banana wore off. No chance of any sneaky sugar from doting grandparents again!

Check your child out on the questionnaire below.

Blood Sugar Check

Does your child...

- [ ] ... usually eat white bread, rice or pasta instead of brown/ wholegrain?
- [ ] ... crave sugar, sweets or refined carbohydrates such as chocolate, biscuits, toast and jam or sweetened cereals?
- [ ] ... have sugary foods or drinks at regular intervals during the day?
- [ ] ... crave caffeinated drinks such as colas?
- [ ] ... sometimes skip meals, especially breakfast?
- [ ] ... seem to be slow to get going in the morning?
- [ ] ... have energy slumps during the day?

☐ ... sometimes lose concentration or have poor attention span?
☐ ... get dizzy, dopey or irritable if he or she doesn't eat often?
☐ ... seem to lack energy?
Tick the box for 'yes'. If you tick five or more, the chances are your child's blood sugar balance is less than perfect.

Later in this chapter we're going to explain exactly what you need to do to improve your child's blood sugar balance and banish these symptoms. Bur first it helps to understand how blood sugar actually works. How does glucose get into the bloodstream, and how do you ensure the right amount ends up there – and reaches your child's brain?

The ups and downs of blood sugar

As we saw above, the raw material of blood sugar are the carbo-hydrates in what you eat and drink. When your child eats carbohydrate-rich foods such as cereal, bread, pasta, potatoes or rice, the sugars and starches in these foods are broken down into glucose during digestion. The glucose is then absorbed into the bloodstream. Some carbohydrates, particularly the refined kind found in white bread, are broken down and absorbed more quickly than others. More on this in a moment.

Refined sugar, technically called sucrose, is the type found in sugary drinks and cereals. Their breakdown and absorption into the bloodstream is even faster, because sucrose and glucose are almost the same thing.

When your child consumes a lot of fast-releasing carbohy-drate all at once (say, in a fizzy drink and biscuits, or white toast and jam), their blood glucose levels will soar. Glucose is powerful stuff, and can actually damage nerves and blood vessels. The body copes with this by enlisting the help of the hormone insulin, which is released from the pancreas when a burst of glucose hits your child's bloodstream.

Once in the blood, insulin escorts the glucose into cells, where it's used for energy. Any excess – and there will be if your child has overdosed on refined carbohydrates – is stored, in a form called glycogen, in other parts of the body such as the muscles and liver. When these stores are full, any remaining glucose is converted to body fat.

In the 'sugar overdose' scenario – after a big bowl of processed, sweetened cereal, say, or a bag of sweets at the cinema – the body responds to what it sees as a dangerous situation by releasing more insulin than normal. As a result, too much glucose can actually be escorted out of the bloodstream, leaving your child with too low a blood glucose level and a subsequent crash in energy. We've seen how nasty the symptoms of low blood glucose can be. But even worse, your child is then likely to crave more of what caused the problem in the first place – sugar – just to get rid of the unpleasant feelings. And round we go again. It's a vicious cycle that leads to more cravings, more extreme mood fluctuations, and progressively poorer concentration and behaviour.

Sugar imbalance and your child

Seesawing blood sugar levels not only affect your child's mood and behaviour; they can also affect their IQ. Research at the Massachusetts Institute of Technology in the US found a massive 25 per cent difference between the IQ scores of children who were in the top fifth of the population for consumption of sugar and other refined carbohydrates, compared with children who were in the bottom fifth.[10] So staying away from white bread, processed cereals and sugar seems to be crucial to having a higher IQ.

But that's not all. To maximise mental performance, your child needs to have that all-important even supply of glucose to the brain. This has been well proven by Professor David Benton at Swansea University, who has found that dips in blood glucose are directly associated with poor attention, poor memory and aggressive behaviour.[11] Sugar has been implicated in aggressive behaviour,[12–17] anxiety,[18–19] hyperactivity and attention deficit,[20] depression,[21] eating disorders,[22] fatigue[23] and learning difficulties.[24–27]

More, dietary studies consistently reveal that hyperactive children eat more sugar than other children,[28] and that reducing dietary sugar has been found to halve disciplinary actions in young offenders.[29] A study of 265 hyperactive children found that more than three-quarters displayed abnormal glucose balance.[30]

Inside carbohydrates

We all need carbohydrates, and they're very important for your child. But as the evidence shows, you need to be choosy about which types they eat. Foods with complex carbohydrates, such as wholegrains, vegetables, beans or lentils, or with simpler carbohydrates such as fruit, take longer to digest than refined carbohydrates. As a result, the glucose released from these foods doesn't flood into the bloodstream, but trickles in slowly over time. This means that it's used for energy rather than stored, leaving blood glucose levels on an even keel, and preventing dramatic changes in mood, behaviour and energy.

Why refined is bad

There's another reason why 'whole' foods, such as whole oats, are better for you than foods rich in refined carbohydrates, such as white bread or pasta. By overprocessing carbohydrate foods, we are cheating nature, isolating the sweetness in the food and discarding the rest.

The most extreme example is concentrated sugar – white sugar, brown sugar, malt, glucose, honey and syrup. These are 'fast-releasing', triggering a rapid rise in blood glucose levels, and at the same time, almost completely devoid of vitamins and minerals. White sugar, for instance, loses up to 90 per cent of the vitamins and minerals present in the raw materials (such as beet sugar) from which it was made. (More on the importance of vitamins and minerals in Chapter 6.)

What about fruit sugar?

The main sugar in most fruit is the simple sugar fructose. This enters the bloodstream fast, but is classified as 'slow-releasing' because the body has to convert it to glucose before it can be used as fuel, and this process slows down its effect on the body.

Some fruits, such as grapes and dates, contain almost pure glucose, putting the carbs they contain in the fast-releasing class. Apples, on the other hand, contain mainly fructose and so are classed as slow-releasing. Bananas contain both, and raise blood glucose levels quite speedily. But all fresh fruit has two big advantages. One is fibre, which slows down the release of the sugars contained in the fruit. The other is vitamins, which as we'll see in Chapter 6 are essential for physical and mental health.

What about dried fruit? In a nutshell, it's problematic. This is because, weight for weight, it obviously has much less water than fresh fruit, and this both concentrates the sugar and makes it much smaller and less filling – so you can end up packing away quite a lot of it without realising. More, the fibre in dried apples, for instance, is less effective at slowing down sugar release. So don't make dried fruit a substitute for fresh. And when you do give your kids dried fruit, soak it first – when it's plumped up and rehydrated it will be more filling, so they're likely to eat less of it.

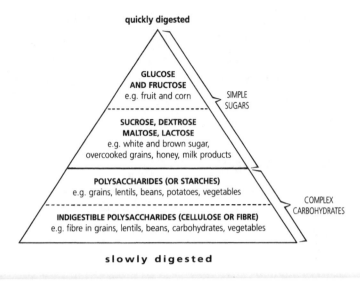

The sugar family

The carbs that keep blood sugar even

Now that we know how important the release rate of carbo-hydrates is, how can you tell which is fast-releasing and which slow? As a general rule, you can assume that whole, unprocessed foods are the slowest to release their sugar. Beyond this, you can use a measure called Glycemic Load (GL) which measures the effect of a food on blood glucose levels. Foods with a GL of less than ten are good and should be the staple foods of your child's diet. A GL of 11 to 14 can be eaten in moderation. A GL higher than 15 should be avoided. Beware of combining two moderate-GL foods in one meal. When they're eaten together, their GL adds up to high. For example, a crumpet with unsweetened peanut butter (moderate with low GL) remains moderate, while the GL score of a crumpet with a teaspoon of honey (moderate with moderate) shoots up.

The chart below gives the GL score of an average serving of a range of common foods. You can start to use this now by checking out what your child eats for breakfast.

If they start the day with puffed rice cereal and raisins, both of which have a high GL score, they're getting rocket fuel first thing in the morning – and that means that a couple of hours later their blood glucose, and energy, will plummet. But give them oat flakes, sweetened with a chopped apple – both of which are slow-releasing – and their energy and concentration will last right through to lunch.

Glycemic Load of Common Foods

Food	Serving size in g	Looks like	GLs per serving
BAKERY PRODUCTS			
Low-carb muffin	–	1 muffin	5
Apple and almond cake	–	1 medium slice	5
Carrot and walnut cake	–	1 medium slice	5
Muffin – apple, made without sugar	60	1 muffin	9
Muffin – apple muffin, made with sugar	60	1 muffin	13
Crumpet	50	1 crumpet	13
Muffin – apple, oat, sultana, made from packet mix	50	1 muffin	14
Muffin – bran	57	1 muffin	15
Banana cake, made without sugar	80	1 medium slice	16
Muffin – blueberry	57	1 muffin	17
Muffin – banana, oat and honey	50	1 muffin	17
Croissant	57	1 croissant	17
Doughnut	47	1 plain doughnut	17
Sponge cake, plain	63	1 slice	17
Muffin – carrot	57	1 muffin	20
BREADS			
Volkenbrot wholemeal rye bread	20	1 slice	5
Rice bread, high-amylose	20	1 small slice	5
Rice bread, low-amylose	20	1 small slice	5
Wholemeal rye bread	20	1 thin slice	5
Wheat tortilla (Mexican)	30	1 tortilla	5
Chapatti, white wheat flour, thin, with green gram	30	1 chapatti	5
Rye kernel (pumpernickel) bread	30	1 slice	6

Food	Serving size in g	Looks like	GLs per serving
Sourdough rye bread	30	1 slice	6
White, high-fibre bread	30	1 thick slice	9
Wholemeal (wholewheat) wheat flour bread	30	1 thick slice	9
Gluten-free fibre-enriched bread	30	1 thick slice	9
Gluten-free multigrain bread	30	1 slice	10
Light rye bread	30	1 slice	10
White wheat flour bread	30	1 slice	10
Pitta bread, white	30	1 pitta	10
Wheat flour flatbread	30	1 slice	10
Gluten-free white bread	30	1 slice	11
Corn tortilla	50	1 tortilla	12
Middle Eastern flatbread	30	1 slice	15
Baguette, white, plain	30	1/9 baton	15
Bagel, white, frozen	70	1 bagel	25
CRISPBREADS/CRACKERS			
Rough Oat Cakes (Nairn's)™	10	1 oat cake	2
Fine Oat Cakes (Nairn's)™	9	1 oat cake	3
Cheesey Oat Cakes (Nairn's)™	8	1 oat cake	3
Cream cracker	25	2 biscuits	11
Rye crispbread	25	2 biscuits	11
Water cracker	25	3 biscuits	17
Puffed rice cakes	25	3 biscuits	17
DAIRY PRODUCTS AND ALTERNATIVES			
Plain yoghurt (no sugar)	200	1 small pot	3
Non-fat yoghurt (plain, no sugar)	200	1 small pot	3
Soya yoghurt (Provamel)	200	1 large bowl	7
Soya milk (no sugar)	(250ml)	1 glass	7
Low-fat yoghurt, fruit, sugar (Ski)	150	1 small pot	7.5
FRUIT AND FRUIT PRODUCTS			
Blackberries	120	1 medium bowl	1
Blueberries	120	1 medium bowl	1
Raspberries	120	1 medium bowl	1
Strawberries, fresh, raw	120	1 medium bowl	1
Cherries, raw	120	1 medium bowl	3
Grapefruit, raw	120	1/2 medium	3
Pear, raw	120	1 medium	4

Food	Serving size in g	Looks like	GLs per serving
Melon/cantaloupe, raw	120	1/2 small	4
Watermelon, raw	120	1 medium slice	4
Peaches, raw (or canned in natural juice)	120	1	5
Apricots, raw	120	4 apricots	5
Oranges, raw	120	1 large	5
Plum, raw	120	4	5
Apples, raw	120	1 small	6
Kiwi fruit, raw	120	1	6
Pineapple, raw	120	1 medium slice	7
Grapes, raw	120	16	8
Mango, raw	120	1 1/2 slices	8
Apricots, dried	60	6 apricots	9
Fruit cocktail, canned (Del Monte)	120	Small can	9
Papaya, raw	120	Half a small papaya	10
Prunes, pitted	60	6 prunes	10
Apple, dried	60	6 rings	10
Banana, raw	120	1 small	12
Apricots, canned in light syrup	120	1 small tin	12
Lychees, canned in syrup and drained	120	1 small tin	16
Figs, dried, tenderised (Dessert Maid)	60	3	16
Sultanas	60	30	25
Raisins	60	30	28
Dates, dried	60	8	42

JAMS/SPREADS

Pumpkin seed butter	16	1 tbsp	1
Peanut butter (no sugar)	16	1 tbsp	1
Blueberry spread (no sugar)	10	1 dessertspoon	1
Apricot fruit spread, reduced sugar	10	1 dessertspoon	2
Orange marmalade	10	1 dessertspoon	3
Strawberry jam	10	1 dessertspoon	3

SNACK FOODS (SAVOURY)

Eggs (boiled)	–	2 medium	0
Cottage cheese	120	1/2 medium tub	2
Egg mayonnaise	120	1/2 medium tub	2
Hummus	200	1 small tub	6
Olives, in brine	50	7	1

Food	Serving size in g	Looks like	GLs per serving
Peanuts	50	2 medium handfuls	1
Cashew nuts, salted	50	2 medium handfuls	3
Potato crisps, plain, salted	30	1 small packet	7
Popcorn, salted	25	1 small packet	10
Pretzels, oven-baked, traditional wheat flavour	30	15	16
Corn chips, plain, salted	50	18	17
SNACK FOODS (SWEET)			
GoodCarb™ Real Belgian Chocolate Brownie (all 3 flavours)	45	1 bar	3
Fruitus apple cereal bar	35	1	5
Euroviva Rebar fruit and veg bar	50	1	8
Apricot fruit bar (dried apricot filling in wholemeal pastry)	35	1	12
Muesli bar with dried fruit	30	1	13
Chocolate bar, milk, plain (Mars/Cadbury/Nestlé)	50	1	14
Twix® biscuit and caramel bar (Mars)	60	1 bar (2 fingers)	17
Snickers® bar (Mars)	60	1	19
Polos peppermint sweets (Nestlé)	30	16	21
Jelly beans, assorted colours	30	9	22
Kellogg's Pop-Tarts™, double choc	50	1	24
Mars Bar®	60	1	26

A comprehensive list of the GL of foods is available in the New Optimum Nutrition Bible *and* The Holford Low-GL Diet, *or online at www.holforddiet.com.*

How to keep your child in perfect balance

As you can see abundantly in the chart above, the GL of some foods is through the roof – and bound to play havoc with your child's blood sugar balance. You may have had a few shocks: baguettes and bagels have quite a high GL, for instance. But as you'll discover, it's amazingly easy to find delicious and thoroughly satisfying substitutes. Here are some examples of what your child should and should not be eating to keep his or her blood glucose level and brain in good balance:

INSTEAD OF...	EAT
White toast and jam	Wholegrain toast and baked beans
Cornflakes	Porridge with berries
Croissants and baguettes	Wholegrain rye breads
White rice	Wholemeal spaghetti
Chocolate bars	Raw vegetable crudités
Bananas	Berries, apples or oranges
Crackers or rice cakes	Oatcakes

Part 4 shows you how to do this in more detail. Now, let's look at what should be on your child's plate – and what needs to stay on the supermarket shelves.

Sugar – the long goodbye

Weaning your child off sugar is a big part of the switch to brain-friendly eating. It's easiest for all concerned to decrease the sugar content of your child's diet slowly and gradually over time, so that he or she will get used to less sweetness without noticing it too much.

For example, sweeten cereal with fruit. Dilute fruit juices with water by at least half to halve their GL score (see page 33 for more advice on juices). Avoid foods with added sugar. Limit dried fruit, and cut down on fast-releasing, high-GL fruits like bananas – or combine them with slow-releasing, low-GL carbohydrates such as oats.

The one exception to this rule is if your child has just done some intense exercise, such as playing a game of football. They'll need to boost their blood sugar levels fast, as not only are their blood sugar levels low, but the glycogen storage facilities in the muscles and liver will also be empty. So there is no harm in their snacking on a fast-releasing fruit such as a banana: any excess glucose in the blood will go to replenish the empty glycogen storage facilities rather than build up into high blood sugar.

Stay away from sugar substitutes

While they won't raise blood sugar levels, sugar substitutes shouldn't be part of your plan to cut down on sugar in your child's diet. Aspartame, the most widely used, is particularly bad. Plenty of studies have shown it to have adverse effects on health in children. One study into the effects of aspartame showed that it caused nightmares, memory loss, temper and nausea.[31] Besides the dangers of additives, there is another good reason not to use them. And that is that they don't help children adjust to less sweet food. For all of us, adults and children alike, staying away from sugar becomes easier and easier as our cravings for sugar subside. Artificial sweeteners simply keep those cravings alive.

One sugar substitute worth a mention is xylitol. It is derived from a natural source and is abundant in plums, which have a very low GL as a result. Xylitol has a fraction of the effect on blood sugar compared with regular sugar or even fructose. For example, 7 teaspoons of xylitol has the same effect on the blood sugar as 4 teaspoons of fructose or 1 teaspoon of sugar. We still suggest you reduce your child's taste for sweet foods, but when some sweetness is really essential, for example, if you're whipping up dessert for a special-occasion meal, then xylitol is the best alternative to sugar. See Resources, page 282, for details of suppliers.

Dynamic duo – protein and fibre

The more fibre and protein you include with any meal or snack, the slower the release of the carbohydrates. Fibre does the job by actually getting in the way of the carbohydrate, impeding its interaction with digestive enzymes and effectively slowing its passage into the intestines where it is absorbed into the bloodstream. Meanwhile, protein slows down the speed at which the stomach empties its contents of partially digested food into the intestines.

As we've seen, anything that slows the passage of carbohydrate into the bloodstream is good for blood glucose balance. So combining protein-rich foods with high-fibre carbohydrates is an excellent rule of thumb in this context. Here's how you do it:

- Give seeds or nuts with a fruit snack

- Add seeds or nuts to carbohydrate-based breakfast cereals

- Serve salmon, chicken or tofu with brown basmati rice

- Add kidney beans to pasta sauce served over wholemeal pasta

- Put cottage cheese on oatcakes, or hummus on rye bread

- Make sandwiches with sugar-free peanut butter and wholemeal bread.

Is it really juice?

Much of the 'fruit juice' on the market is not much better than sugary water. Once a fruit juice has been processed and put into a carton, it bears little resemblance to a fresh fruit juice in terms of colour, taste and nutrient content.

Unfortunately, however, the sugar content remains intact. Children who regularly drink processed juice are taking in a lot of sugar, and thereby messing up their blood glucose balance, feeding their sugar cravings and rotting their teeth. Despite vigorous marketing to convince us to the contrary, the stuff in these cartons is not a good source of vitamins and minerals. Worst of all are the 'juice drinks'– these almost invariably have added sugars and very little actual fruit juice.

This doesn't mean juice is completely off the menu. You

simply need to go for freshly squeezed. Or failing that, chill-cabinet juices, which are obviously fresher; just be vigilant about checking labels to discover the shelf life. If this is longer than just a few days into the future, we recommend you don't touch it. If it is expected to 'go off' in a few days, then it was probably reasonably nutritious when it went into the carton, but its nutrient content is declining by the hour. So inevitably, fruit that's juiced right in front of you is the best bet.

Along with freshness, you need to look at the GL score of various juices. Apple and pear are best, followed by orange. As we mentioned above, it's also important to dilute the juice your child drinks 50/50 with water, as this halves the GL score. Fresh vegetable juices can be drunk without dilution, with the possible exception of carrot juice.

Don't go without breakfast

Getting the kids up on a school morning with enough time for them to eat a decent breakfast can be challenging at the best of times. But eating a decent breakfast really is essential for your child to be able to concentrate at school. If their blood sugar stays rock-bottom all morning, they'll experience all the problems we've mentioned, from dizziness to a lack of mental focus.

In one study, 29 schoolchildren were given different breakfast cereals, a glucose drink or no breakfast on different days. Their attention and memory were tested before breakfast, and again 30, 90, 150 and 210 minutes later. Children who had had the glucose drink or no breakfast showed poorer attention and memory compared to the children eating cereal.[32]

We find that children who eat a nutritious diet generally get a much better night's sleep, too (see Chapter 24). The knock-on effect is that it's easier for them to get out of bed in the morning – which in turn gives them the time and inclination to eat a decent breakfast.

If your child doesn't have much of an appetite in the

morning and frequently skips breakfast, help them by easing them into the habit gradually. Begin by giving them one strawberry. The next day, make it two strawberries and a brazil nut or a teaspoon of sunflower seeds. The next day, half an apple and three almonds – and so on until after a couple of weeks they'll be able to eat a bowl of oats (as porridge, or raw as muesli) with fruit and nuts. Remember that you too need to eat breakfast! If you typically go to work on a cup of coffee, don't be surprised if your children attempt to imitate you in their own way.

Stay off the caffeine

Sugar isn't the only factor in blood sugar problems. Stimulants are too – and as caffeine is a powerful one, it can be highly disruptive to your child's blood sugar balance. Caffeine is also an appetite suppressant, and as such can be implicated in behaviours like picky eating or refusing to contemplate breakfast.

Supermarket shelves groan with products containing caffeine. Let's look at the biggest culprits.

Cola and energy drinks These contain anything from 46 to 80mg of caffeine per can – as much as you'd find in a regular cup of filter coffee. These drinks are often also high in sugar and colourings, and their net stimulant effect can be considerable. Check the label on all canned drinks, and keep your children away from any that contain caffeine and chemical additives or colourings. Also watch out for 'natural' stimulants like guarana: these have the same effect as caffeine.

Chocolate bars and drinks Chocolate is everywhere these days, along with hordes of chocoholics. The bars are usually full of sugar, which is bad enough for blood glucose levels, but cocoa, the active ingredient in chocolate and in chocolate drinks, also provides significant quantities of the stimulant theobromine. Theobromine's action is similar to caffeine's, though not as strong. Chocolate also contains small amounts of caffeine.

As chocolate is high in sugar and stimulants, reserve it as a special treat for your child. That means a small amount once a week rather than every day. Also bear in mind the relative size of the chocolate bar and your child. For example, don't give a toddler more than a square or two of chocolate at one sitting.

Tea Some people start their children off on the great British addiction very young indeed. Yet a strong cup of tea contains as much caffeine as a weak cup of coffee and is certainly addictive. Tea also contains tannin, which interferes with the absorption of vital minerals such as iron and zinc. Even 'decaffeinated' tea is not actually caffeine-free, it simply has reduced caffeine and the tannin levels remain the same.

If you want to give your child a hot drink, the best alternatives to tea are Rooibosch tea (red bush tea) with or without milk, and herbal or fruit teas. Since these are naturally caffeine-free, they have no downsides.

Coffee Coffee is fast overtaking tea as the number one hot drink of the nation and again, many children are taking up the habit at a young age. Coffee contains three stimulants – caffeine, theobromine and theophylline. Although caffeine is the strongest of the three, theophylline is known to disturb normal sleep patterns and theobromine has a similar effect to caffeine's, although it is present in much smaller amounts in coffee.

So there's a host of stimulants in coffee waiting to mess up your child's blood sugar balance. But that's not all. It is also addictive, and despite general public perception, it actually worsens mental performance. Research published in the *American Journal of Psychiatry* studied 1,500 psychology students and found that moderate and high consumers of coffee were found to have higher levels of anxiety and depression than abstainers, and that the high consumers had the greatest incidence of stress-related medical problems, as well as lower academic performance.[33] A number of studies have shown that the ability to remember lists of words is made worse by caffeine, so children who drink coffee before school, especially as a pre-exam boost, are more likely to struggle in class.

The reason people get hooked on caffeine, particularly in the morning, is that it makes you feel better, more energised and alert. However, Dr Peter Rogers, a psychologist at Bristol University, wondered whether caffeine actually increases your energy and mental performance, or just relieves the symptoms of withdrawal.

When he researched this he found that, after that sacred cup of coffee, coffee drinkers don't feel any better than people who never drink coffee – they just feel better than they did when they woke up.[34] In other words, drinking coffee relieves the symptoms of withdrawal from caffeine. So the important message here is – don't let your children start drinking coffee. It isn't good for them, and like any addiction, giving up becomes more difficult the longer you have the habit.

Like decaffeinated tea, **decaffeinated coffee** isn't stimulant-free because only some of the caffeine is removed and the other stimulants remain. The most popular alternatives are Teeccino, Caro, Barley Cup, dandelion coffee or herbal teas. If your child already has the taste for coffee, offer a choice of these substitutes. They may experience 'withdrawal' symptoms when they give up coffee, such as headaches, but these will disappear within a few days.

In summary, here are some general guidelines to ensure your child's brain gets an even supply of glucose.

- **Choose wholefoods – wholegrains, lentils, beans, nuts, seeds, fresh fruit and vegetables. With fruit and veg, go for dark green, leafy and root vegetables such as watercress, carrots, sweet potatoes, broccoli, Brussels sprouts, spinach, green beans or peppers, raw or lightly cooked. Choose fresh fruit such as apples, pears, berries, melon or** citrus fruit and, infrequently, bananas. Provide five or more servings of fruits and vegetables each day.

- Avoid overly processed foods.

- Choose wholegrains such as rice, buckwheat, millet, rye, oats, wholewheat, corn or quinoa in cereal, breads and pasta. Avoid refined 'white' foods.

- Avoid sugar and foods containing sugar. This means anything with added glucose, sucrose and dextrose. Keep fructose consumption within limits. Don't be tempted to go for sugar substitutes – most are detrimental to health and they all keep sugar cravings alive.

- Combine protein foods with carbohydrate foods by giving cereals and fruit with nuts or seeds, and ensuring your child eats carbohydrate-rich foods (potato, bread, pasta, or rice) with protein-rich foods such as fish, chicken, lentils, beans or tofu. As fibre is important for slowing sugar absorption, make sure your child is getting ample fibre in fruit and veg.

- Choose real fresh fruit juices from the chill cabinet and dilute 50/50. Steer clear of the highly processed kind with a long shelf life.

- Encourage your child to eat breakfast.

- Help your child avoid caffeinated food and drinks, such as chocolate, tea and coffee.

CHAPTER 3

Smart Fats - The Mind's Construction Crew

 We humans are fatheaded: the solid part of our brains is a good 60 per cent fat. In a child, this fatty tissue is constantly growing and maintaining itself, so a good supply of the raw materials – essential fats – is needed to build a healthy brain. These aren't just any old fats, and it's vital that your child gets the right kind, in the right quantities.

Three-year-old Adrian is a case in point. His parents brought him to see us at the Brain Bio Centre because they were concerned about his loss of speech development. They had already put him on a dairy and gluten-free diet and were pleased to see that his eczema disappeared and his asthma had improved dramatically. We ran some tests which showed he was very low in magnesium, selenium and zinc and also in essential fats. We recommended supplementation of fish oils and a multivitamin and mineral. Within days of starting the fish oil, Adrian began to chatter again.

Check your child out on the questionnaire below.

Fat Check

....

Does your child...

☐ ... eat oily fish (salmon, trout, sardines, herring, mackerel or fresh tuna) less than once a week?

☐ ... eat seeds or their cold-pressed oils fewer than three times a week?

☐ ... eat meat or dairy products most days?

☐ ... eat processed or fried foods (such as ready meals, chips or crisps) three or more times a week?

☐ ... have dry or rough skin or a tendency to eczema?

☐ ... have dry or dull hair or dandruff?

☐ ... suffer from dry, watery or itchy eyes?

☐ ... suffer from excessive thirst or frequent urination?

☐ ... have frequent mood swings?

☐ ... have a poor memory, attention span or difficulty concentrating?

☐ ... have poor physical coordination?

Tick the box for 'yes'. If you tick five or more, the chances are your child isn't getting enough essential fats. By upping your child's intake, these symptoms can rapidly improve.

....

We'll be explaining later in this chapter how to dramatically boost your child's essential levels with the right food and supplements. But first, let's look more closely at what they do.

Essential fats – miracle in mind

Essential fats – the omega-3 and omega-6 essential fats – help children stay physically healthy, reducing the risk of allergies, asthma, eczema and infections. More than this, they promote mental health. A deficiency can result in depression, dyslexia, attention deficit disorder, autism, fatigue, memory and behaviour problems. The bottom line is that essential fats really *are* essential for keeping the state of your child's brain in healthy equilibrium. And these fats are also needed in optimal amounts to maximise your child's intelligence.

We use the word 'intelligence' very broadly here. Your child's ability to perform in this world depends upon a balance of mental, emotional and physical intelligence. Mental intelligence we are very well aware of, because of IQ tests that determine a person's ability to make intellectual connections and deal with complex concepts.

But emotional intelligence is no less important. Your child's EQ is a measure of his or her ability to respond emotionally to situations in an appropriate and sensitive way. If they lose their temper easily, and oscillate between depression and hyperactivity, lacking emotional balance and perspective, there's room for improvement – however 'bright' they may be.

Then there's physical intelligence. PQ is all about brain-body coordination. For example, a lot of children diagnosed with attention deficit disorder are clumsy by nature (with or without a diagnosis of dyspraxia), and have trouble with skills such as handwriting, reading and taking notes in class.

Never too late to start

Every type of intelligence – IQ, EQ and PQ – is affected by your child's intake of the omega-3s and omega-6s. Children deficient in essential fats have more learning difficulties, while children who are breastfed have higher IQs at age eight than bottle-fed babies, which is thought to be due to the higher levels of essential fats in breast milk.[35] [36]

Recent studies by Dr Peter Willatts at the University of Dundee in Scotland showed that babies fed a formula enriched with a specific omega-3 essential fat (DHA) had better problem-solving skills at ten months of age.[37] Also, supplementation of omega-3 essential fats to women while pregnant and breastfeeding has been shown to improve their child's intellectual function right up to their fourth year.[38] Research is underway that is likely to show that these benefits persist into adulthood.

Essential fats remain essentially important throughout life, so your child will continue to need it as they grow – and beyond. The good news is that it's never too late to boost your child's essential fat levels so that they can reap the benefits.

For example, research by Dr Alex Richardson at Oxford University has proven the value of essential fats in a 'double-blind' trial involving 41 children aged 8 to 12 years who had symptoms of ADHD and specific learning difficulties. Those children receiving extra essential fats in supplements were both behaving and learning better within 12 weeks.[39] Another trial by Dr Richardson showed significant improvement in reading ability in children on essential fat supplements, compared with children taking a placebo, over six months.[40]

All this confirms American surveys carried out at Purdue University that show children with ADHD tend to get lower levels of essential fats than children without ADHD.[41] Supplementation with these was found to reduce ADHD symptoms such as anxiety, attention difficulties and general behaviour problems.[42–44]

So, while it seems such a simple thing, giving your child an essential fat supplement can have profound benefits for their mental abilities.

How omegas do the job

All the evidence points to essential fats as vital to the ongoing task of keeping your child in good mental health. In fact, the brain and nervous system totally depend on them, and never more so than during pregnancy and childhood. The other important fat families are saturated and monounsaturated fats and cholesterol. Your child's brain contains vast amounts of cholesterol, for instance, and it is used to make the sex hormones oestrogen, progesterone and testosterone. But these fats can be made in the body. The omega fats have to be supplied through diet, which is why you need to ensure your child's level of them stays topped up.

To fully understand what omega fats do in the brain, let's take a closer look at a neuron.

As we saw in Chapter 1, intelligence – and the process of thought itself – involves the careful connecting up of billions of nerve cells, each one of which links to thousands of others. You'll remember that the 'messengers', neurotransmitters, deliver their messages across connection points called synapses into receptor sites.

These receptor sites are contained within the myelin sheath, which surrounds every neuron in the brain. The sheath is a bit like a layer of insulation around an electrical wire. Without it, the transmission of messages – and thus, the working of the brain – would be impossible. The sheath is roughly 75 per cent fat, and it's here that the omegas have a starring role.

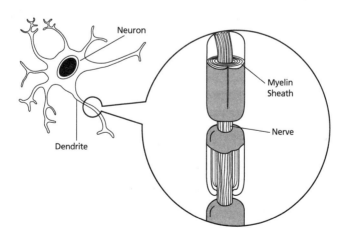

Close-up of a neuron

Myelin sheath fat is made out of phospholipids (more on these in the next chapter), each with a saturated and unsaturated fatty acid attached. In the figure below you'll see the unsaturated fatty acid as a bent squiggle. This is most often an omega-3 or omega-6 fat.

Both kinds of omega fats need to be in balance – in fact, this balance seems to be critical for the smooth working and restructuring of the brain. So for brain health, you'll need to supply both omega-3 and omega-6 fats in your child's diet.

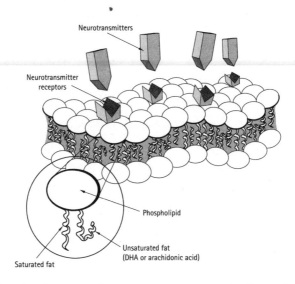

The myelin sheath surrounding neurons is composed of phospholipids and fats

Omega-3 and 6 in your child's diet

Despite all the evidence in favour of essential fats, many adults and increasingly more children are 'fat phobic', and may shy away from taking them. The reason is that all types of fat are generally lumped together – and fat gets a lot of bad press.

Some of this is deserved. The damaged or hydrogenated

(solidified) fats found in processed or fried foods and some margarines are bad for health, yet they're everywhere – as are saturated fats in dairy products and meat. As a result, most people in the West are eating too much of them.

But this doesn't mean you need to put your child on a low-fat diet. You just need to ensure that the fats in their diet are the right kind – the omegas. If your child is concerned that eating them will lead to weight gain, you should know that they can actually help with weight loss! So even if your child is over-weight, he or she should still be eating essential fats, while cutting down on the saturated fats in meat and dairy, and completely cutting out the 'trans' fats found in fried and processed foods. (Chapter 23 will tell you what to look for on labels to avoid these fats.)

Most of us are deficient in the omega fats, particularly in omega-3s, as we will see. And many children are grossly deficient, as the many child health problems related to deficiency show. Ultimately, however, the most precise way to know your child's essential fat status is to have a blood test. This is what we do at our London-based Brain Bio Centre, and they're also available through other nutritional therapists. The test gives you a complete breakdown of all the essential fats, and shows which ones are lacking.

Fat figures

How much essential fat will your child need to stay mentally and physically healthy? To answer that, we first need to look at the optimal amount of overall fat in their diet.

It is best to consume no more than 20 per cent of all calories as fat. The current average in Britain is around 40 per cent. In countries with a low incidence of fat-related diseases such as heart disease, like Japan, Thailand and the Philippines, people consume only about 15 per cent of their total calorie intake as fat.

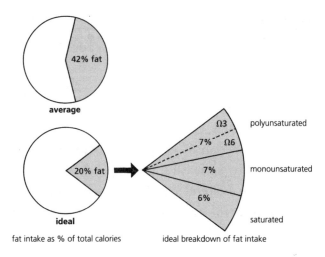

What we eat vs what we need

Most authorities now agree that of our total fat intake, no more than a third should be saturated fat, and at least a third should be polyunsaturated oils providing the two essential fats, omega-3 and omega-6. As we saw earlier, these two essential fat families also need to be roughly in balance – in a ratio of 1:1, which is what our ancestors were getting before the Industrial Revolution. Then, people ate local foods with an abundance of seeds, whereas the widespread exodus to the cities resulted in the rise of easily stored refined foods and hard fats. So nowadays, the average balance is more like 1:20 in favour of omega-6s.

So it may not just be the gross deficiency in omega-3 fats that has led to so many of the health problems we're seeing in children today, but also the gross imbalance between the two omegas. In addition, a high intake of saturated fats and the damaged polyunsaturated fats we call trans fats stop the body from making good use of the little essential fat the average person does eat in a day.

The omega-3s

By now you'll have gathered how important the omega fat families are to your child's mental and emotional health. Let's delve deeper, first taking a closer look at the essential fats so many children lack – the omega-3s.

Why is the modern-day diet likely to be more deficient in omega-3 fats than in omega-6s? It's all because the grandmother of the omega-3 family, alpha-linolenic acid, and her metabolically active grandchildren EPA (eicosapentaenoic acid) and DHA (docosahexaenoic acid), are more unsaturated and so more prone to damage by cooking, heating and food processing. For example, if you fry a piece of fish or roast seeds, you will actually damage some of the omega-3s they contain. In any event, the average person today eats a mere sixth of the omega-3 fats found in the average European diet of 1850. This decline is partly due to food choices, but mainly due to food processing.

Alpha-linolenic acid, the omega-3 'grandmother', is abundant in cold climate seeds, such as flaxseeds, and also plankton – the vegetation of the sea. Our bodies can convert some of this alpha-linolenic acid into EPA and DHA, but a more effective way to increase supplies of these more 'active' omega-3s is to eat oily fish.

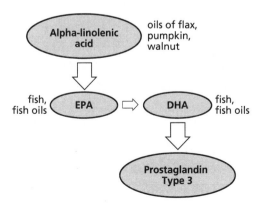

Omega-3 fat family

This is because the fish has already effectively done the conversion for us in its own body. The primary source of EPA and DHA is coldwater fish, especially fish that eat fish – namely herring, mackerel, salmon and fresh tuna. Sardines are also an excellent source.

There are a few caveats here. Since canned tuna has much less omega-3, stick with fresh tuna. But as larger fish like tuna tend to be higher in mercury, don't feed tuna steaks to your child more than two or three times a month week, and less if they show signs of mercury toxicity (more on this in Chapter 7). As for salmon, the amount of EPA and DHA in the farmed fish really depends on the quality of its diet, and as with most intensive farming practices this can be variable. Organic farmed or wild salmon is much better in this respect.

As a rule of thumb, children normally need around 300 to 400mg of both DHA and EPA a day (see Chapter 26 for supplement levels for different age ranges). The conversion in the body of alpha-linolenic acid in, say, flax (linseeds) and pumpkin seeds, to EPA and DHA can be very inefficient. For this reason vegetarians rarely have sufficient levels of EPA and DHA unless they eat significant quantities of flaxseeds, which are the richest source of alpha-linolenic acid.

So during critical periods of development such as childhood, it may be preferable to get a direct source of EPA and DHA from fish, backed up by an indirect supply from flaxseeds or flaxseed oil. This would certainly be recommended for a pregnant or breastfeeding woman to allow her to pass on sufficient EPA and DHA to her child. The World Health Organization now recommends that formula feeds include these oils.[45] DHA is especially important during the foetal stage and infancy because it is literally used to build the brain, and makes up a full quarter of the brain's dry weight.

In many cases, children with learning and behavioural problems are even less efficient than the average at converting alpha-linolenic acid into EPA and DHA. Partly for this reason, a child with ADHD or dyslexia may need double or triple their intake to correct their condition.

The best diet from the point of view of omega-3 fats is a 'fishitarian' one where your child eats fish three times a week; or, failing that, a seed-rich vegan diet. Eggs can also provide significant quantities of omega-3 if the hens were fed a high-omega-3 diet – check the eggbox labels.

Remember: not only is it important to eat a direct source of omega-3 fats such as fish or a rich, indirect source such as flaxseeds. It's also vital for your child to eat less saturated and processed fat. We'll see why in a bit.

The omega-6s

Your child will also need omega-6 fats. Of all the tissues of the body, the brain has the highest proportion of these fats.

The grandmother of the omega-6 fat family is linoleic acid, which is found in seeds, especially hot-climate seeds such as sunflower and sesame seeds. Linoleic acid is converted by the body into gamma-linolenic acid (GLA), which may be familiar to you as a substance in evening primrose oil and borage or starflower oil, the richest known sources. A derivative of GLA, known as DGLA, is found in high quantities in the brain.

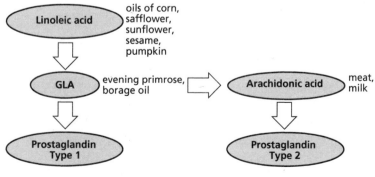

Omega-6 fat family

Supplementing GLA, usually from evening primrose oil, has proven effective in alleviating a wide variety of mental health problems. For example, a study on children with dyspraxia showed that supplementation with essential fats including omega-6 oil improved reading, writing and behaviour in just three months.[46]

One omega-6 fat has something of a Jekyll and Hyde nature, however, and that's arachidonic acid (AA). While there is no question that it is essential for brain function, arachidonic acid is bad news in excess in the body, as it is associated with promoting inflammation. It can be derived either directly from meat or animal produce, or indirectly from linoleic acid or GLA. The latter may be a preferable source because GLA also produces anti-inflammatory substances that balance the inflammatory effects of arachidonic acid.

For this and other reasons, it's best to let your child eat omega-6-rich seeds and their oils to get enough of this essential fat family, rather than overdosing on meat and dairy produce.

Where to get the omegas

As we've seen, the seeds with the highest levels of omega-3 fats are flax. Hemp and pumpkin seeds are rich sources, too. The only direct source of the essential omega-3 brain boosters EPA and DHA are oily fish.

The best seeds for omega-6 fats are hemp, pumpkin, sunflower, safflower, sesame and maize kernels. Walnuts, soya beans and wheatgerm are also rich in omega-6s.

Best Foods for Brain Fats

OMEGA-3	OMEGA-6
Flaxseeds (linseed)	Corn
Hempseed	Safflower
Pumpkin seeds	Sunflower
	Sesame
	Walnut

EPA & DHA	GLA
Salmon	Evening primrose oil
Mackerel	Borage oil
Herring	Blackcurrant seed
Sardines	
Anchovies (whole, not salted fillets)	
Tuna steak	
Eggs (of flaxseed-fed hens)	

So what's the best way of incorporating these essential fats into your child's daily menu? There are three possibilities: seeds and fish; seed oils, which are more concentrated in essential fats but don't provide other nutrients such as minerals, which are abundant in the whole seeds; or supplementing concentrated fish oils and seed oils such as flax, evening primrose or starflower oil.

Now let's look at how to put those ideas into practice.

Seeds and fish If you want to go with seeds, put one measure each of sesame, sunflower and pumpkin seeds, and three measures of flaxseeds, into a sealed jar.

Keep it in the fridge, away from light, heat and oxygen. Simply adding one heaped tablespoon of these seeds, freshly ground in a coffee grinder, to your child's breakfast each morning guarantees a good daily intake of essential fats. We'd also recommend that your child eats 100g of oily fish (roughly equivalent in size to one tin of sardines or a mackerel fillet) two or three times a week.

Seed oils If you want to go with oils, the best place to start is an oil blend that offers a 1:1 ratio of omega-3 and omega-6 fats, is cold-pressed, preferably organic and kept refrigerated before you buy it. These are now widely available in health food stores (see Resources, page 280). The oil can be added to salads and other cold or warm foods, but must not be heated. Some children will take it neat off the spoon.

Hempseed oil is the next best thing. It provides 19 per cent alpha-linolenic acid (omega-3), 57 per cent linoleic acid and 2 per cent GLA (both omega-6s). Chapter 26 gives details of supplement levels for different age ranges.

Supplements As far as supplements are concerned, for omega-6 your best bet is starflower (borage) oil or evening primrose oil. Starflower oil provides more GLA and fish oils are best for omega-3. There are supplements that combine EPA, DHA and GLA. For smaller children who can't swallow supplements, there are a number of supplements in liquid form and flavoured in various ways. Levels of these to supplement are discussed in detail in Chapter 26.

Fats to avoid or limit

The kind of fat your child eats alters the fat composition in his or her brain. If it's the omega or other fats that were there in the first place, all is well; but if it's the fats that so much junk and other processed foods are riddled with, your child will be rebuilding his or her brain with fats that fail to manage the brainwork required of them.

Trans fat – the worst culprit

The worst fats your child can eat are the trans fats we've talked about – damaged fats found in deep-fried food and foods containing hydrogenated vegetable oils. To minimise your child's exposure to trans fats, limit their intake of fried and especially deep-fried food, and don't buy foods containing hydrogenated fats. Check the list of ingredients in processed foods: if a food has the word 'hydrogenated' in the ingredients, don't put it in your basket. Another clue is shelf life. Trans fats are widely used to extend shelf life, so a long shelf life is a warning sign that the food probably contains trans fats and/or preservatives.

Why are trans fats so bad for your child? They can be taken directly into the brain and appear in the same position as DHA in brain cells, where they proceed to make a hash of the information-processing job DHA does so brilliantly. Trans fats also block the conversion of essential fats into vital brain fats such as GLA and DHA. Twice as many trans fats appear in the brains of people deficient in omega-3 fats.

So a combined deficiency in omega-3 fats and an excess of trans fats – the hallmark of the chicken-nugget-and-fries generation – is a bad scenario. A serving of chips or fried fish can each deliver 8g of trans fats, a doughnut 12g, and a bag of crisps more than 4g. The ideal amount in your child's diet is zero.

Saturated and monounsaturated fats

Saturated fats are typically solid at room temperature, and include butter, cheese, lard (the fat in meat) and coconut oil. While you don't want your child to eat large amounts of saturated fat, a small amount is fine. One good use of these fats is for frying. Saturates are not damaged by heat and converted into trans fats in the way that the polyunsaturates such as the omega fats are. So we suggest using butter or virgin coconut oil if you're frying food at home. Always fry at the lowest possible temperature to reduce the amount of oxidants you create (more on this in Chapter 24).

Monounsaturated fats, which include olive oil, are liquid at room temperature but will start solidifying if refrigerated (the omega fats and other polyunsaturates remain liquid even at much lower temperatures). There is plenty of research to show that good-quality olive oil contributes to health, making it perfect for salad dressings.

Cholesterol

Similar to saturated fats, a moderate amount of cholesterol in the diet is perfectly acceptable and even necessary. How good or bad it is depends on how it's cooked. Overcooked, fried or burnt cholesterol is bad for your child's health, so don't fry eggs or bacon until they are crispy, or char meat.

In summary, here are some general guidelines to ensure your child gets enough brain fats.

- **Provide plenty of seeds and nuts – the best seeds are flax, hemp, pumpkin, sunflower and sesame. You get more goodness out of them by grinding them first and sprinkling on cereal, soups and salads.**

- **Choose coldwater carnivorous fish – a serving of sardines, mackerel, herring, kipper or wild/organic salmon two or three times a week provides a good source of omega-3 fats.**

- **Choose cold-pressed seed oils – either an oil blend or hemp oil for salad dressings and other cold uses.**

- **Avoid fried food and processed food.**

- **Choose fish oil to supplement omega-3 fats, and starflower or evening primrose oil for omega-6 fats.**

CHAPTER 4

Phospholipids – Go to School on an Egg

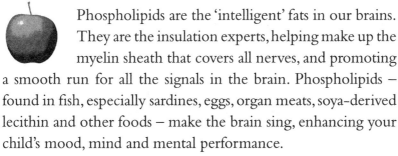 Phospholipids are the 'intelligent' fats in our brains. They are the insulation experts, helping make up the myelin sheath that covers all nerves, and promoting a smooth run for all the signals in the brain. Phospholipids – found in fish, especially sardines, eggs, organ meats, soya-derived lecithin and other foods – make the brain sing, enhancing your child's mood, mind and mental performance.

Check your child out on the questionnaire below.

Phospholipid Check

Does your child...

☐ ... eat fish less than once a week?

☐ ... eat fewer than three eggs per week?

☐ ... eat soya/tofu or nuts less than three times per week?

☐ ... take less than 1g of lecithin in supplements or granules each day?

☐ ... have a poor memory?

☐ ... find it hard to do calculations in his/her head?

☐ ... sometimes have difficulty concentrating?

☐ ... have a tendency toward depression?

☐ ... appear to be a 'slow learner'?

Tick the box for 'yes'. If you tick five or more, the chances are your child isn't getting enough phospholipids.

....

Superbrains in the making?

There are two kinds of phospholipids – phosphatidyl choline and phosphatidyl serine, otherwise known as PC and PS. Supplementing these smart fats as well as eating foods rich in choline and serine, from which they're built, has some very positive benefits for your child's brain. Let's look at choline first.

Choline – memories are made of this

To give you some idea of just how dramatic the effect of choline on the brain can be, consider this study from Duke University Medical Center in North Carolina in the US. During the study, researchers demonstrated that giving choline during pregnancy creates the equivalent of super-brains in rat offspring.

The team fed choline to female rats halfway through their pregnancy. The infant rats whose mothers had been fed the choline had vastly superior brains with more neuronal connections, and consequently, improved learning ability and better memory recall, all of which persisted into old age. In essence, this research shows that giving choline helps restructure the brain for improved performance.[47] And although the focus was on rats, we would expect a similar effect in humans.

Choline's starring role in mental performance is down to the fact that it is the direct source of acetylcholine, the memory neurotransmitter in our brains. In fact, choline deficiency is a common cause for poor memory.

Supplementing choline not only makes more acetylcholine.[48] It also goes to form a vital building material for nerve cells and the receptor sites for neurotransmitters. According to Professor Richard Wurtman of the Massachusetts Institute of Technology, if your choline levels are depleted, your body grabs the choline that you need to build your nerve cells to make more acetylcholine.[49] So Wurtman believes that providing the brain with enough of this vital brain nutrient is essential.

PS: don't forget the phosphatidyl serine

Phosphatidyl serine, sometimes known as the memory molecule, is a smart nutrient that can genuinely boost your child's brainpower. The secret to the memory-boosting properties of PS is probably due to its ability to help brain cells communicate, as it is a vital part of the structure of the brain's receptor sites.

The positive effects of supplementing PS are just as amazing as those of supplementing choline. We've seen children with learning problems make enormous progress just by adding in a source of these vital phospholipids.

Eat your phospholipids

Although we can make phospholipids in the body, getting some extra from dietary sources is even better.

The richest sources of phospholipids in the average diet, as we've seen, are eggs and organ meats. This explains why lions and other animals at the top of the food chain eat the organs and brain first – they're not stupid! You can also find choline in soya beans, peanuts and other nuts.

But nowadays, as the number of children suffering from memory and concentration problems soars, our intake of phospholipids is sinking dramatically. For example, to top up our dietary PS to the level of about 50mg a day, we'd have to eat a lot of liver and other organ meats – not a very likely scenario these days. Vegetarians are unlikely to achieve even 10mg of PS a day.

A daily supplement can really help some children's memories – see Chapter 26 for details of amounts for different age ranges. Phospholipids are often a part of brain food formulas. And there are other ways of getting these wonder fats back into your child's diet – let's look at them now.

Rediscover the egg

Eggs are delicious, as well as the richest source of choline and an excellent source of PS. But people these days are often egg-phobic, thinking that they are an unhealthy food due to their high fat and cholesterol content. This just isn't true. As we learnt in the last chapter, some fat and cholesterol are essential for health.

The kind of fat you find in an egg depends on what you feed the chicken. If you feed them a diet rich in omega-3s, for example flaxseeds or fishmeal, you get an egg high in omega-3s. An egg is as healthy as the chicken that laid it.

As for cholesterol, it is simply a myth that what you find in eggs is bad for you or your child – it will neither raise blood cholesterol nor cause heart disease. And as long as you don't fry it, a free-range, organic, omega-3-rich egg is a veritable super-food. Go for lightly boiled or hardboiled eggs, poached eggs or gently scramble them; you can safely give your child six to ten eggs a week.

Lecithin – gold in those granules

Lecithin is the best source of phospholipids, and is widely available in health food shops, where it's sold either as lecithin granules or capsules. The easiest and cheapest way to take this is to add a tablespoon of lecithin, or a heaped teaspoon of high-

PC (phosphatidyl choline) lecithin, to your child's cereal in the morning.

And in case you were wondering, lecithin won't make your child fat. In fact, quite the opposite: it helps the body break down fat.

In summary, here are some general guidelines to help ensure your child has an optimal intake of phospholipids.

- Add a tablespoon of lecithin granules, or a heaped teaspoon of high-PC lecithin, to your child's cereal every day.

- Or give your child an egg for breakfast – preferably free-range, organic, high in omega-3s and lightly boiled, poached or scrambled, but definitely not fried.

- Or supplement a brain food formula providing phosphatidyl choline and phosphatidyl serine, especially if your child is having learning problems. See Chapter 26 for details.

CHAPTER 5

Protein – The Architect of Mind and Mood

 Protein provides amino acids – the building blocks of life. Just as a sentence is made up of words, and words of letters, protein is made up of peptides and peptides are made up of amino acids.

When your child eats protein-rich foods such as meat, eggs, fish, dairy, lentils, beans or quinoa (an Andean grain, pronounced 'keen-wa'), his or her digestive system breaks down the protein first into peptides and then into amino acids. By linking these amino acids together in different sequences, their body then builds up new muscle or organ tissue or neuro-transmitters – the chemical messengers of the brain. So a good supply of protein, and hence of amino acids, will keep your child's brain running super-smoothly.

Deficiency in amino acids isn't at all uncommon and can give rise to depression, apathy and lack of motivation, an inability to relax, poor memory and concentration. But supplementing specific amino acids has been proven to correct all these problems. For example, a form of the amino acid trypto-phan has proven more effective in double-blind trials than the best antidepressant drugs,[50] the amino acid tyrosine improves mental and physical performance under stress better than coffee,[51] and the amino acid GABA is highly effective against anxiety.[52]

Amino Acid Check

Does your child...

- [ ] ... eat less than one portion of protein-rich foods (meat, dairy, fish, eggs, tofu) each day?
- [ ] ... eat fewer than two servings of vegetable sources of protein (beans, lentils, quinoa, seeds, nuts, wholegrains and so on) each day?
- [ ] ... if they're vegetarian, do they rarely combine different protein foods such as those mentioned above?
- [ ] ... engage in a lot of physical activity?
- [ ] ... suffer from anxiety, depression or irritability?
- [ ] ... seem to be frequently tired or lack motivation?
- [ ] ... sometimes lose concentration or have poor memory?
- [ ] ... grow slowly or have slow-growing hair and nails?
- [ ] ... seem to be constantly hungry?
- [ ] ... frequently get indigestion?

Tick the box for 'yes'. If you tick five or more, the chances are your child isn't getting enough amino acids. Upping their intake of protein can make all the difference.

Read on to discover how to boost your child's protein intake and boost their mental and physical energy. But to understand why amino acids are so important for your child's brain, we first need to explore what the neurotransmitters they build actually do.

Key players in the orchestra of mind

There are hundreds of different kinds of neurotransmitters in the brain and body, but here are the main players:

- **Adrenalin, noradrenalin and dopamine** make us feel good, stimulating us, motivating us and helping us deal with stress

- **GABA** counteracts these stimulating neurotransmitters, by relaxing us and calming us down after stress

- **Serotonin** keeps us happy, improving our mood and banishing the blues

- **Acetylcholine** keeps our brain sharp, improving memory and mental alertness

- **Tryptamines** keep us connected. For example, melatonin keeps us in sync with day and night and the seasons.

Many other substances in the brain act much like neurotransmitters, such as endorphins, which give us a sense of euphoria after exercise, for example. But the ones above are the big five – the key players in the orchestra. And your child's mood, memory and mental alertness are all affected by their activity.

If serotonin is up, for example, your child is likely to be happy; if dopamine and adrenalin are down, he or she is likely to feel unmotivated and tired. Having the right balance of these key neurotransmitters is a must if you want your child to be in tip-top mental health, and supplementing the right amino acids can solve a wide variety of mental health problems in children.

And how do the amino acids do the job? Their action is very similar to that of prescribed drugs that directly affect neurotransmitters. For instance, amphetamines such as Ritalin work by causing an excessive release of adrenalin, whereas antidepressants like Seroxat effectively raise levels of serotonin by preventing its breakdown in the body. But these drugs have many undesirable side-effects, essentially working against our body's natural design, not with it. And antidepressants such as Seroxat are also falling out of favour, particularly regarding use in children, as more and more studies show the benefits do not outweigh the risks.

Nutrients such as amino acids work just as well, if not better, but don't have the side-effects: after all, it's part of the brain and body's natural design to use them. So the best way to tune up your child's brain is to ensure they have an adequate intake of amino acids in their diet. First and foremost, this means eating enough protein every day.

Power of protein

The quality of a protein is determined by its balance of amino acids. Though there are 23 amino acids from which the body can build everything, from a neurotransmitter to a muscle cell, only eight are known as essential – because they only come through diet. The other 15 can be made in the body from the essential eight if there is not enough of them in the diet. The better the balance of amino acids – expressed as a unit called an NPU, which stands for 'net protein usability' – the more you can make use of the protein.

The chart overleaf shows the top 24 individual foods and food combinations in terms of NPUs, or protein quality. Combining lentils or beans with rice, for example, is a great way of increasing the overall quality of the protein because the amino acids rice is low in, lentils and beans are rich in. It also shows how much of a food, or food combination, you need to eat to get a 20g serving of protein. A child needs to eat between one or two of these servings a day, depending on their age (see below).

Protein Requirement by Age

	2–3 years	4–8 years	9–13 years	14–18 years (girls)	14–18 years (boys)
Protein (g)	13	19	34	46	52

A typical day's protein for a six-year-old might therefore include two of any of the following: an egg (10g), a 50g serving of salmon, a handful (60g) of seeds and nuts, or a serving of beans (100g).

For a vegetarian child, a typical day's worth might be any two of the following: a small tub of yoghurt, a handful of seeds or nuts, a 140g (5oz) serving of tofu, a small cup of quinoa, or a small serving of beans with rice. The trick for vegetarians is to eat 'seed' foods – that is, foods that would grow if you planted them, which includes seeds, nuts, beans, lentils, peas, quinoa maize or the germ of grains such as wheat or oat. 'Flower' foods such as broccoli or cauliflower are also relatively rich in protein.

Note that the cup measures indicated are Imperial.

Packed with Protein: The Top 24			
Food	**Percentage of calories as protein**	**Amount needed to provide 20g (¾oz) protein**	**Protein quality (NPU)**
Grains/Pulses			
Quinoa	16	100g (3.5oz)/1 cup dry weight	Excellent
Tofu	40	275g (10oz)/1 packet	Reasonable
Maize	4	500g (1lb 2oz)/3 cups cooked weight	Reasonable
Brown rice	5	400g (14oz)/3 cups cooked weight	Excellent
Chickpeas	22	115g (4oz)/0.66 cup cooked weight	Reasonable
Lentils	28	85g (3oz)/1 cup cooked weight	Reasonable
Fish/meat			
Tuna, canned	61	85g (3oz)/1 small tin	Excellent
Cod	60	35g (1.25oz)/1 very small piece	Excellent
Salmon	50	100g (3.5oz)/1 small piece	Excellent
Sardines	49	100g (3.5oz)/1 baked	Excellent
Chicken	63	75g (2.5oz)/1 small roasted breast	Excellent
Nuts/seeds			
Sunflower seeds	15	185g (6.5oz)/1 cup	Reasonable
Pumpkin seeds	21	75g (2.5oz)/0.5 cup	Reasonable
Cashew nuts	12	115g (4oz)/1 cup	Reasonable
Almonds	13	115g (4oz)/1 cup	Reasonable

Food	Percentage of calories as protein	Amount needed to provide 20g (¾oz) protein	Protein quality (NPU)
Eggs/dairy			
Eggs	34	115g (4oz)/2 medium	Excellent
Yoghurt, natural	22	450g (1lb)/3 small pots	Excellent
Cottage cheese	49	125g (4.5oz)/1 small pot	Excellent
Vegetables			
Peas, frozen	26	250g (9oz)/2 cups	Reasonable
Other beans	20	200g (7oz)/2 cups	Reasonable
Broccoli	50	40g (1.5oz)/0.5 cup	Reasonable
Spinach	49	40g (1.5oz)/0.66 cup	Reasonable
Combinations			
Lentils and rice	18	125g (4.5oz)/small cup dry weight	Excellent
Beans and rice	15	125g (4.5oz)/small cup dry weight	Excellent

Be aware, though, that your child can have too much protein: more doesn't always mean better. Once daily protein intake goes above 85g a day (depending on your child's current growth pattern, exercise level and hence requirement) this can have negative health consequences.

For instance, the breakdown products of protein, such as ammonia, are toxic to the body and stress the kidneys during elimination. Also, too many amino acids mean too much acid in the blood, which the body neutralises by releasing calcium from bone. It is now well established that diets very high in protein contribute to kidney disease and osteoporosis. So, as with all else in nutrition, balance is important.

Supplementing amino acids

If your child is eating a reasonable amount of protein (and chewing it thoroughly), he or she should be getting all the amino acids that he or she needs. But if he or she is having particular problems with mood or memory, you can consider supplementation (more on this in Part 3). Tests to measure levels of amino acids in the blood are available through nutritional therapists (see Resources, page 278), who may then recommend supplementation of particular amino acids based on the results.

In summary, here are some general guidelines to help ensure your child has an optimal intake of amino acids.

- Give them between one and two servings of the protein-rich foods shown in the table above every day, depending on their age.

- Include some protein with every meal, such as chickpeas or chicken in their pasta sauce or nuts and seeds with their cereal.

- Choose good vegetable protein sources, including beans, lentils, quinoa, tofu (soya) and 'seed' vegetables such as broccoli.

- If your child is eating animal protein, choose free-range eggs, fish or lean meat, and go for organic whenever possible.

CHAPTER 6

Why Vitamins and Minerals Make Your Child Brainy

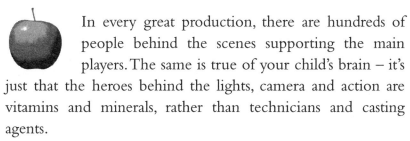 In every great production, there are hundreds of people behind the scenes supporting the main players. The same is true of your child's brain – it's just that the heroes behind the lights, camera and action are vitamins and minerals, rather than technicians and casting agents.

One of the main roles of vitamins and minerals is to help turn glucose into energy, amino acids into neurotransmitters, simple essential fats into more complex fats like GLA or DHA, and choline and serine into phospholipids. They are key to the task of building and rebuilding the brain and nervous system, and keeping everything running smoothly.

Since we have long known they're essential for your child's brain, back in the early 1980s we decided to test what would happen to the intelligence of schoolchildren if given an optimal intake of vitamins and minerals. Gwillym Roberts, a schoolteacher and nutritional therapist from the Institute for Optimum Nutrition, and Professor David Benton, a psychologist from Swansea University, devised a test putting 60 schoolchildren onto a special multivitamin and mineral supplement designed to ensure an optimal intake of key nutrients.[53]

But without their knowledge, half these children took a placebo.

After eight months on the supplements, the non-verbal IQs in those taking the supplements had risen by over ten points! No changes were seen in those on the placebos. This study, published in *The Lancet* in 1988, has since been proven many times in other studies. Most have used RDA levels of nutrients, which are much lower than those in our original study, but still show increases in IQ averaging 4.5 points.

Why do vitamins and minerals raise IQ? The answer appears to be that children think faster and can concentrate for longer with an optimal intake of vitamins and minerals. Check your child out on the questionnaire below.

Intelligent Nutrient Check

Does your child...

☐ ... eat fewer than five servings of fresh fruits and vegetables (excluding potato) every day?

☐ ... eat fewer than one portion of a dark green vegetable a day?

☐ ... eat fewer than three portions of fresh or dried tropical fruit a week?

☐ ... eat seeds or seed oils (such as pumpkin, sunflower, tahini) or unroasted nuts less than three times a week?

☐ ... typically not take a multivitamin/mineral supplement?

☐ ... usually eat white bread, rice or pasta instead of brown/whole-grain?

☐ ... suffer from anxiety, depression or irritability?

☐ ... suffer from muscle cramps?

☐ ... have white marks on more than two fingernails?

☐ ... seem disconnected and find it difficult to relate or communicate?

Tick the box for 'yes'. If you tick five or more, the chances are your child isn't getting enough vitamins and minerals.

The ultimate head start

The dividends of giving your child the vitamins and minerals they need right from the start are enormous. That means during pregnancy (and ideally, before conception), while breastfeeding and also during the weaning process.

A 16-year study by the Medical Research Council shows just how critical optimum nutrition is in the early years. They fed 424 premature babies either a standard or an enriched milk formula containing extra protein, vitamins and minerals. At 18 months, those fed standard milk 'were doing significantly less well' then the others, and at eight years old had IQs up to 14 points lower.[54]

In Chapter 21 we give you details on how to keep your growing child optimally nourished through pregnancy and early infancy. But remember: it's never too late to increase brain-boosting vitamins and minerals in your child's diet, as you will see later.

Nutrients for brain vitality

Every one of the 50 known essential vitamins and minerals plays a major role in promoting mental health. In the chart below we list the most vital to the state of your child's brain, along with the symptoms you might see if your child is deficient, and the best food families to feed your child to ensure they get enough.

Key Vitamins and Minerals for Brain Health		
Nutrient	**Symptoms of Deficiency**	**Food Source**
B1	Poor concentration and attention	Wholegrains, vegetables
B3	Depression, psychosis	Wholegrains, vegetables
B5	Poor memory, stress	Wholegrains, vegetables

Nutrient	Symptoms of Deficiency	Food Source
B6	Irritability, poor memory, depression, stress	Wholegrains, bananas
Folic acid	Anxiety, depression, psychosis	Green leafy vegetables
B12	Confusion, poor memory, psychosis	Meat, fish, dairy products, eggs
Vitamin C	Depression, psychosis	Vegetables and fresh fruit
Magnesium	Irritability, insomnia, depression, hyperactivity	Green vegetables, nuts, seeds
Manganese	Dizziness, convulsions	Nuts, seeds, tropical fruit
Zinc	Confusion, blank mind, depression, loss of appetite, lack of motivation and concentration	Oysters, nuts, seeds, fish

Other vitamins and minerals affect brain health indirectly: antioxidants, for instance, offer protection from pollution, while minerals keep depression, confusion and insomnia at bay. We'll look at them all in more detail – but first, a glance at the B family of vitamins.

The B vitamins

B vitamins are absolutely key to mental health in all of us, children and adults alike. The brain uses a huge amount of them, and as they're water-soluble and pass rapidly out of the body, even a short-term deficiency in any one of the eight Bs can result in a rapid shift in how your child thinks and feels. So it's best for them to get a regular intake throughout the day.

As you saw from the chart, this shouldn't be difficult: a healthy, balanced diet is rich in the foods rich in Bs. The best sources of B1, B3, B5 and B6 are wholegrains and vegetables (B6 is abundant in bananas, too), while to keep folic acid topped up you'll need to provide plenty of spinach and other green leafy veg, and for B12 you'll need good protein such as eggs and fish.

While the deficiency symptoms of B vitamins are well known, we still do not know exactly why many of them occur. Each B vitamin has so many functions in the brain and nervous system that there are few hard proofs in this regard. But we do know one of the best indicators of deficiency – homocysteine levels (see Box).

B deficiencies – the homocysteine link

How do you know if your child is getting enough B vitamins? One of the best gauges is homocysteine, a toxic protein found in the blood. If your child's levels of blood homocysteine are high, they are likely to be low in B6, B12 or folic acid because these vitamins help get rid of homocysteine. So they'll need to top up their Bs.

Because of this intimate inverse link between homocysteine and Bs, and the importance of Bs to brain health, your child's homocysteine level can be seen as a measure of their biological IQ.

To demonstrate this, researchers from Örebro University in Sweden compared school grades in 10 core subjects with homocysteine levels in a group of 692 school children aged 9 to 15. They found that higher homocysteine levels were strongly associated with lower grades.[55]

The ideal level of blood homocysteine for an adolescent or adult is below 7μmol/l. For a child of 10 or younger, the level should ideally lie below 5μmol/l. See the resources section (page 278) for details of how to get your child tested, and Chapter 26 for details on supplementation to bring a high homocysteine level down into the ideal range.

Vitamin B1 (thiamine)   Vitamin B1 helps turn glucose, the brain's main fuel, into energy – so one of the first symptoms of thiamine deficiency is mental and physical tiredness.

Children low in this vitamin have a poor attention span and concentration.

David Benton, professor of psychology at the University of Swansea, one of the leading experts in nutrition and IQ, has found that low levels of thiamine correlate with poor cognitive function in young adults. His research results also show that thiamine supplementation was associated with reports of feeling more clearheaded, composed and energetic and having faster reaction times, even in those whose thiamine status, according to the traditional criterion, was adequate.[56–57]

Vitamin B3 (niacin)   Of all the nutrients connected with mental health, niacin or vitamin B3 is the most well-known. Niacin is recognised as crucial to blood glucose balance, and in the manufacture of both serotonin (the 'happy' neurotransmitter) and melatonin (the sleep enhancer) from the amino acid tryptophan. Thus it is important in keeping your child on an even emotional and mental keel, in good spirits, and sleeping well at night.

Vitamin B5 (pantothenic acid)   Pantothenic acid or B5 is a potent memory booster. It is needed to make the memory-boosting neurotransmitter, acetylcholine. Supplementing extra B5, particularly with choline, can definitely sharpen your child's memory (see Chapter 12).

Vitamins B6, B12 and folic acid   This trio, together with riboflavin (B2), control a critical process in the body called methylation, which is vital in the formation of almost all neurotransmitters. Abnormal methylation lies behind many mental health problems, as we'll find out later in this book. A lack of B6, for example, means we don't make serotonin so efficiently, which could potentially lead to depression. B6 can help relieve stress too, while stress depletes B6. So, if your child is B6 deficient and stressed, he or she may be heading for depression.

Vitamin B12 is vital for a healthy nervous system. Without this crucial nutrient, neither the senses nor the brain can work properly. Even slightly low B12 levels have been linked to poor mental performance in adolescents.[58]

Getting enough B6, B12 and folic acid is absolutely vital in pregnancy too, both for protecting against developmental problems such as spina bifida and for general mental development. Children born to mothers deficient in folic acid show delayed intellectual development.[59]

As you'll have gathered, these nutrients have so many critical roles to play in the brain and nervous system that ensuring your child is getting optimal levels is really a prerequisite for mental health.

Antioxidants – protecting your child's brain

We live in a highly polluted world, and there may not be a lot you can do to avoid many of the pollutants. But you can protect your child's brain from the inside, with antioxidants.

Antioxidants are the antidote to oxidants, also known as 'free radicals' – highly unstable molecules that can trigger cellular damage. They are a byproduct of normal body processes and of combustion. In the body, oxidants are produced every time glucose is 'burnt' within a cell to make energy, and they can go on to damage the essential fats, proteins and phospholipids that make up your child's brain and nervous system. In the environment, they can result from, say, a car's burning of petrol as fuel and emerge in the exhaust.

If we see oxidants as the sparks from something burning, such as food frying or a smoking cigarette, antioxidants are like fire-proof gloves that prevent the sparks from damaging your brain.

A single puff of a cigarette contains a trillion oxidants, which rapidly travel into the brain. This is why smoking around children is especially bad news. Less avoidable are the oxidants from exhaust fumes, particular diesel. These have an insidious effect on your child's body and brain – and that is why it's crucial for your child to have a good intake of antioxidants.

Most important for the brain is the fat-based antioxidant vitamin E. This prevents the chain reactions of damage caused when oxidants enter the brain. Vitamin E is properly called 'd-alpha tocopherol', and its relatives gamma-tocopherol and tocotrienols are also important for the brain. These are only found in the better-quality supplements that contain vitamin E together with 'mixed tocopherols'. They are also present in vitamin E-rich foods, such as seeds, cold-pressed seed oils, fish and avocados.

There are other vital antioxidants. Vitamin C, for example, helps 'recycle' vitamin E once it has grabbed hold of an oxidant. Of course, vitamin C does much more than protect your child from pollution. It has many roles to play in the brain, such as helping to balance neurotransmitters.

Among the many members of this fire-fighting team, the main ones are shown in the figure below showing how the body detoxifies an oxidant from fried food.

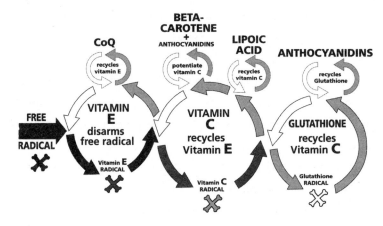

How antioxidants disarm an oxidant or 'free radical'

To give your child maximum protection, it's worth making sure their daily supplement contains antioxidants, as well as giving them foods high in them, such as:

- **Beta-carotene** – carrots, sweet potatoes, dried apricots (soaked first), squash, watercress

- **Vitamin C** – broccoli, peppers, kiwi fruit, berries, tomatoes, citrus fruit

- **Vitamin E** – seeds and their cold-pressed oils, wheatgerm, nuts, beans, fish, avocados

- **Selenium** – oysters, Brazil nuts, seeds, molasses, tuna, mushrooms

- **Glutathione** – tuna, pulses, nuts, seeds, garlic, onions

- **Anthocyanidins** – berries, cherries, red grapes, beetroot, prunes

- **Lipoic acid** – red meat, potatoes, carrots, yams, beets, spinach

- **Co-enzyme Q** – sardines, mackerel, nuts, seeds.

But be aware that maximising your child's mental powers isn't just about what your child eats. It's also about what he or she doesn't eat. As well as the oxidants we all make just from burning glucose as fuel, eating a piece of crispy meat introduces millions of these culprits. So it is important not to overcook, burn or char food. A barbecue is great fun, but do cook on lower flames and ensure your children's sausages are gently browned and cooked all the way through – not charred black on the outside. If you like to fry food, try sautéing it gently on low heat with the lid on the pan. If the oil spits or smokes in the frying pan, it's too hot.

Mineral marvels

Vitamins get a lot of the good press, but certain minerals are key to brain health, helping your child calm down, grow and get through puberty with less stress – to name just a few benefits. Let's look at them now.

Calcium and magnesium   Giving children a mineral may be the last thing you'd think of doing to calm and relax them and help them sleep. Yet that's precisely what calcium and magnesium do, by helping to relax nerve and muscle cells.

Muscle cramps are an obvious sign of magnesium deficiency. A lack of either calcium or magnesium can also make children more nervous, irritable and aggressive. Magnesium has been used successfully to treat autistic and hyperactive children, together with other nutrients. Most of all, it helps them to sleep.

Magnesium is typically the second most commonly deficient mineral after zinc (see below) in children. Green, leafy vegetables are rich in it because it is part of the chlorophyll molecule, which gives plants their green colour. So are nuts and seeds, particularly sesame, sunflower and pumpkin. An ideal intake of magnesium is probably 500mg a day, which is almost double what most people achieve. But it's not hard to do: a tablespoon of seeds a day, plus 100mg in a multimineral, is a good way to ensure your child is getting enough.

Zinc   The most commonly deficient mineral, and one of the most critical nutrients for mental health, is zinc. This is particularly true for children since zinc is necessary for growth. A deficiency in this mineral is associated with hyperactivity, autism, depression, anxiety, anorexia, schizophrenia and delinquency – in short, it's implicated in a huge range of mental health problems. Yet the average intake in Britain is 7.5mg, which is half the RDA of 15mg – and means half the British population get less than half the level of zinc thought to protect against deficiency.

Zinc has several crucial roles to play in brain development and maintenance, not least the prevention of oxidation and the synthesis of serotonin and melatonin.[60] Even healthy 'normal' children appear to benefit from extra zinc, as demonstrated in North Dakota in the US recently. Researchers gave zinc supplements to 209 seventh-grade children, aged 10 to 11. They found that those taking 20mg of zinc a day had faster, more accurate memory retrieval and better attention spans within three months than those taking 10mg (the US RDA) or a placebo.[61]

There are also many times during their development when children need a boost from extra zinc: growth spurts, puberty, stress, infections, excess copper, blood sugar problems and even an inherited need for more of this mineral. Boys need extra zinc from about age 12, as zinc in their bodies is concentrated in sperm. Sure signs of zinc deficiency are stretch marks, white spots on the fingernails and teenage acne, an increasingly common phenomenon seen in teenaged girls and boys.

You'll find zinc in any 'seed' food – nuts, seeds and the germ of grains. Meat and fish are rich sources, but none is richer than oysters: a single oyster can provide as much as 15mg of zinc!

Here are a few simple steps you can take to ensure your child gets plenty of vitamins and minerals.

- **Make sure your child eats plenty of foods rich in antioxidants – fruits, vegetables, seeds and fish. Their diet should include at least five, and ideally seven, servings of fresh fruit and vegetables a day.**

- **Serve nuts and seeds daily, and choose wholefoods, such as wholegrains, lentils, beans and brown rice, rather than refined food.**

- **Make sure your child takes an 'optimum nutrition' multivitamin and mineral every day (see Chapter 26 for guidance of the ideal formula depending on your child's age.)**

- **Don't smoke, and keep your kids away from smoky places, to avoid overexposure to oxidants.**

CHAPTER 7

Don't Let Your Child be a Heavy Metal Kid

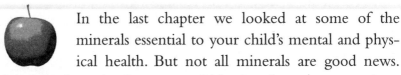 In the last chapter we looked at some of the minerals essential to your child's mental and physical health. But not all minerals are good news. Some, such as the 'heavy metals' lead and mercury, are thoroughly bad news if they find their way into your child's brain and nervous system. High intakes of cadmium and mercury can have a disastrous effect on intelligence and behaviour in children and adults alike.

A high intake of heavy metals in children has been associated with mood swings, poor impulse control and aggressive behaviour, poor attention span, depression and apathy, disturbed sleep patterns, impaired memory and intellectual performance. If your child has symptoms like these, we recommend you have them tested for heavy metals. If these are found, you'll need to remove the source and provide the right nutrients to help detoxify your child's mind and body.

Nine-year-old Antony is a case in point. He had been diagnosed with dysgraphia – a learning difficulty that specifically affects handwriting. His parents had already noticed that his writing was directly affected by sugar and E-numbers and had already taken these out of his diet to good effect. We conducted a hair analysis which showed that he had high levels of the toxic metal mercury in his hair. We increased his intake of zinc, selenium and vitamin C to help his body remove the mercury and three months later Antony and his mother were happy to report that he had had a significant improvement in his handwriting.

Here are some examples of heavy metals, the effect they have on mental health, where they originate, and the nutritional protectors that help to lower body levels of them.

ANTI-NUTRIENT	EFFECT	SOURCE	PROTECTOR
Cadmium	Aggression, confusion	Cigarettes	Vitamin C, zinc
Mercury	Headaches, memory loss	Pesticides, fillings, vaccinations	Selenium
Aluminium	Associated with senility	Cookware, water	Zinc, magnesium
Copper	Anxiety and phobia	Water pipes	Zinc
Lead	Hyperactivity, aggression, low IQ	Exhaust fumes	Vitamin C, Zinc

Now let's take a closer look at just what these culprits can do to our children's mental health.

Heavy metals – the usual suspects

You might think you'd only be exposed to heavy metals if you lived or worked near a toxic dumping ground or the like. The shock is discovering how common they are in the environment.

Cadmium – peril as you puff

Cigarette smoke is laden with cadmium, a heavy metal associated with disturbed mental performance and increased aggression. This nasty also lurks in car exhaust fumes and there can be small amounts in food, especially if it's refined. This happens because beneficial minerals that act as cadmium protectors, such as selenium, are taken out during the refining process. Cadmium also knocks out zinc, so passive smokers will need more.

Keep your children away from cigarette smoke. If you smoke, quit – this is the best way to prevent your children from picking up the habit while protecting them from heavy metal contamination.

Aluminium – toxic takeaway

Aluminium is found in a staggering array of modern products. Aluminium trays and foils are widely used as food packaging by supermarkets, fast-food outlets and other food-handling operations, and the stuff also turns up in many common household products. It's in antacids, toothpaste tubes, pots and pans, even our water.

Not all aluminium will enter the body, however. Only under certain circumstances will aluminium leach from a pan, for example. Old-fashioned aluminium cookware, if used to heat something acidic like tea, tomatoes or rhubarb, will leach particles of aluminium into the water. Also, the more zinc deficient you are, the more aluminium you absorb.

To be safe, it's best not to grill food directly on aluminium foil. Instead, use the grill shelf and place the foil underneath the shelf.

Mercury – why hatters were mad

'Mad as a hatter' – the phrase originated in the 18th and 19th centuries, when mercury compounds were used to make felt for hats. When the felt was boiled, then steamed into shape, hatmakers absorbed the mercury-laden fumes. Their 'madness' was all down to mercury's disturbance of brain processes, which can cause depression, irritability, loss of coordination and other distressing symptoms.

This heavy metal is, in fact, very toxic indeed. Small amounts reach us from contaminated foods, pharmaceuticals, cosmetics and amalgam tooth fillings. Mercury has also been used as a constituent of thimerosal, found in diptheria and hepatitis vaccines, although this practice has recently been stopped.

Of particular concern is fish caught in polluted waters. Mercury is used in a number of chemical processes, and accidents and illegal dumping have resulted in a rise in mercury levels in some areas, including the English Channel. Fish, especially larger fish like tuna, swordfish, marlin and shark, store the mercury – and we end up ingesting it if we eat them.

Oily fish such as tuna are a valuable source of omega-3 essential fats, however (see Chapter 3). The chart below lists coldwater fish in terms of the inverse ratio of omega-3s to mercury – with the best having the greatest amount of omega-3 to the lowest amount of mercury. There may be significantly lower amounts of omega-3 in farmed salmon compared to wild salmon because the amount of the essential fat in the fish depends to a large extent on the quality of its diet.

	Omega-3 g/100g	Mercury mg/kg	Omega-3/ mercury
Fresh wild salmon	2.7	0.05	54.0
Canned sardines	1.57	0.04	39.3
Canned and smoked salmon	1.54	0.04	38.5
Fresh mackerel	1.93	0.54	35.7
Herring (kipper)	1.31	0.04	32.8
Trout	1.15	0.06	19.2
Fresh tuna	1.5	0.4	3.8
Cod	0.25	0.11	2.3

	Omega-3 g/100g	Mercury mg/kg	Omega-3/ mercury
Fresh sole	0.1	0.05	2.0
Canned tuna	0.37	0.19	1.9
Marlin (? = guestimate)	?2	1.1	1.8
Swordfish (? = guestimate)	?2	1.4	1.4

The copper controversy

Copper is both an essential mineral and a toxic one. It's rare to be deficient in copper, except in people whose diets are very high in refined foods, largely because of the widespread use of copper water pipes. These leach small amounts of copper into water. However, if you live in a soft-water area or in a house with new copper piping that hasn't yet got calcified, your family can be exposed to toxic levels of copper.

Copper and zinc are enemies. So if your child is zinc deficient, he or she may not be able to get rid of any excess copper.

Lead – trouble in mind

In the 1990s there were a number of important studies that showed consistently lower IQ in children whose blood, hair or baby teeth contained the highest levels of lead. When Herbert Needleman, an associate professor of child psychiatry, conducted a follow-up study of children who had had elevated lead levels 11 years earlier, he found a sevenfold increase in the odds of failure to graduate from high school, lower class standing, greater absenteeism, more reading disabilities, and poor vocabulary, fine motor skills, reaction time and hand-eye coordination.[62]

Fortunately, since the advent of unleaded petrol, lead is much less of a problem these days. Some lead remains in the environment, but the most likely source these days is drinking water from old lead pipes. Symptoms of lead toxicity include lowered IQ, aggression and headaches.

How to handle the heavies

We've seen the problem. Now, how to fix it? First you need to discover which, if any, toxic minerals are affecting your child.

Hair mineral analysis: the heavy metal MOT

There's a simple way to find out if these heavy and toxic minerals are affecting your child – a hair mineral analysis. By analysing a small amount of hair, your child can be effectively screened not only for the bad guys such as lead, cadmium, mercury and aluminium, but also for the good guys such as magnesium, zinc, chromium, manganese and so on. At around £50, it's well worth it.

But what do you do if your child has raised levels of toxic minerals? Luckily, many essential minerals have an antagonistic relationship with heavy metals. This means that taking more of the essential minerals depletes the toxic ones. So once you've done a hair analysis, it's worth seeing a nutritional therapist for tailored advice to detox your child. See Resources on page 278 for details on how to find a nutritional therapist near you.

Foods that fight heavy metals

Meanwhile, you can certainly improve your child's detoxification, if they need it, by following the general nutrition guidelines in this book, ensuring they get plenty of antioxidants from fresh fruits and vegetables and also plenty of water.

In terms of specific foods, there are a few that can help keep your child's brain 'clean'. Garlic, onions and eggs contain sulphur-containing amino acids, specifically methionine and cystine, which protect against mercury, cadmium and lead toxicity. Pectin in apples, carrots and citrus fruits also helps to remove heavy metals – yet another reason for an apple a day!

In summary, here are some general guidelines to help keep your child free from heavy metals.

- Supplement a multivitamin and mineral including zinc, selenium and vitamin C for toxic mineral protection – see Chapter 26 for our specific supplement recommendations.

- Have a hair mineral analysis for your child, available through nutritional therapists (see Resources).

CHAPTER 8

Keeping Your Child Chemical Free

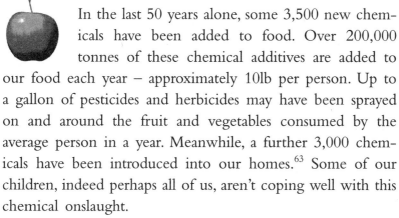In the last 50 years alone, some 3,500 new chemicals have been added to food. Over 200,000 tonnes of these chemical additives are added to our food each year – approximately 10lb per person. Up to a gallon of pesticides and herbicides may have been sprayed on and around the fruit and vegetables consumed by the average person in a year. Meanwhile, a further 3,000 chemicals have been introduced into our homes.[63] Some of our children, indeed perhaps all of us, aren't coping well with this chemical onslaught.

All these compounds are classified as anti-nutrients – substances that interfere either with our ability to absorb or to use essential nutrients, or in some cases, that promote the loss of essential nutrients from the body.

A high intake of anti-nutrient chemicals has been associated with mood swings, poor impulse control and aggressive behaviour, poor attention span, depression and apathy, disturbed sleep patterns, impaired memory and intellectual performance. The best way to remedy or indeed prevent these kinds of symptoms is to keep these chemicals out of your child's diet as much as possible.

Battling the additive blues

For example, tartrazine (E102) is still added into many popular soft drinks for children to colour it yellow/orange, yet has been consistently linked to hyperactivity in children. And in fact, a closer look at this food chemical reveals something rather sinister.

Dr Neil Ward from the University of Surrey decided to test what happens to minerals when drinks containing tartrazine were consumed. He gave children identical-looking and tasting drinks, some with tartrazine and some without. He found that adding tartrazine to drinks increased the amount of zinc excreted in the urine, perhaps by binding to zinc in the blood and preventing it from being used by the body.[64]

In this study, like many others, he also found emotional and be-havioural changes in every child who consumed tartrazine. Four out of the 10 children in the study had severe reactions, three ex-periencing an outbreak of eczema or having an asthma attack within 45 minutes of ingestion. Tartrazine is one of the first of over 1,000 chemical food additives proven to be an anti-nutrient.

Researchers at the University of Southampton investigated the effect of artificial food colourings and a preservative in the diet of 1,873 three-year-old children. They found that the chil-dren's behaviour was worse when the food colourings (a mixture of sunset yellow, tartrazine, carmosine and ponceau 4R) and preservative (sodium benzoate) were in their diet than not. Interestingly, the effect was no different for children who had previously been identified as hyperactive compared with those who were determined not to be hyperactive.[65]

The primary reasons for adding chemicals to food is to make the food look better by changing its colour, and to preserve and stabilise it. Most of the additives are synthetic compounds, some with known negative health effects. But more impor-tantly, we don't know what the long-term consequences of consuming such large amounts of additives are. This is especially true for children whose brains and bodies are still developing. It is therefore best to avoid all additives, with a few notable exceptions. These are:

- The colours E101 (vitamin B2), E160 (carotene, vitamin A)

- The antioxidants E300–304 (vitamin C), E306–309 (tocopherols, like vitamin E)

- The emulsifier E322 (lecithin)

- Stabilisers E375 (niacin), E440 (pectin).

The chart below gives the most up-to-date information on the worst of the food additives. In many cases it's not possible to say with any certainty how these foods might affect your child's mental health.

However, since the brain is not separate from the body, we know that any substance that can have such a negative effect on physical health is likely to have a negative effect on mental and emotional health. There is a distinct lack of research in this area because food manufacturers have no desire to carry out studies beyond the minimum requirements to enable them to put these additives into food.

Top 20 Additives to Avoid

Allura red AC   E129

How used: Widely used as food colouring, in snacks, sauces, preserves, soups, wine, cider, etc.

What you need to know: Avoid if your child has asthma, rhinitis (including hay fever) and urticaria (an allergic rash also known as hives).

Amaranth   E123

How used: Food colour used in jams, jellies and cake decorations.

What you need to know: Banned in the US. Avoid if your child has asthma, rhinitis, urticaria and other allergies.

Aspartame   E951
How used: Widely used as a sweetener in snacks, sweets, desserts, 'diet' foods.
What you need to know: Aspartame may affect people with PKU (phenylketonuria). Recent reports show the possibility of headaches, blindness and seizures with long-term, high-dose aspartame.

Benzoic acid   E210
How used: Widely used preservative in many foods, including drinks, low-sugar products, cereals, meat products.
What you need to know: Can temporarily inhibit the function of digestive enzymes and may deplete glycine levels. Should be avoided by those with allergic conditions such as hay fever, hives and asthma.

Brilliant black BN   E151
How used: Widely used in drinks, sauces, snacks, cheese.
What you need to know: People who suffer from allergic conditions, asthma, rhinitis, urticaria, etc., should avoid this substance.

Butylated hydroxy-anisole (BHA)   E320
How used: Very widely used as a preservative, particularly in fat-containing foods, confectionery, meats.
What you need to know: The International Agency For Research On Cancer say that BHA is possibly carcinogenic to humans. BHA also interacts with nitrites to form chemicals known to be mutagenic (that is, that cause changes in the DNA of cells).

Calcium benzoate   E213
How used: Preservative in many foods, including drinks, low-sugar products, cereals, meat products.
What you need to know: Can temporarily inhibit the function of digestive enzymes and may deplete levels of the amino acid glycine. Should be avoided by those with hay fever, hives and asthma.

Calcium sulphite   E226

How used: Very widely used, mainly as a preservative in a vast array of foods – from burgers to biscuits, and frozen mushrooms to horseradish pulp.

What you need to know: In the US, sulphites are banned from many foods, including meat, because they make old produce look fresh. They can cause bronchial problems, flushing or reddening of the skin, low blood pressure, tingling and anaphylactic shock. The International Labour Organisation (ILO) says to avoid them if you suffer from bronchial asthma, cardiovascular or respiratory problems, or emphysema.

Monosodium glutamate (MSG)   E621

How used: Widely used as a flavour enhancer.

What you need to know: Those sensitive to monosodium glutamate have felt symptoms including pressure on the head, seizures, chest pains, headache, nausea, burning sensations and tightness of face. Many baby-food producers have stopped adding MSG to their products.

Ponceau 4R, Cochineal red A   E124

How used: Widely used as colouring.

What you need to know: People who suffer from asthma, rhinitis, urticaria, may find their symptoms become worse following consumption of foods containing this colouring.

Potassium benzoate   E212

How used: See calcium benzoate (above).

What you need to know: See calcium benzoate (above).

Potassium nitrate   E249

How used: Used as a preservative in cured meats and canned meat products.

What you need to know: Three main health concerns: it can lower the oxygen-carrying capacity of the blood; it may combine with other substances to form nitrosamines, which are carcinogenic; and it may have an atrophying effect on the adrenal gland.

Propyl p-hydroxy-benzoate, propyl-paraben, paraben   E216

How used: Preservatives in cereals, snacks, pate, meat products and confectionery.

What you need to know: Parabens have been identified as the cause of chronic dermatitis in numerous instances.

Saccharin and its Na, K and Ca salts E954
How used: Very widely used sweetener, found in diet and no-added-sugar products.
What you need to know: The International Agency For Research On Cancer has concluded that saccharin is possibly carcinogenic to humans.

Sodium metabisulphite E223
How used: Widely used as a preservative and antioxidant.
What you need to know: May provoke life-threatening asthma – a woman developed severe asthma after eating a salad with a vinegar-based dressing containing E223.

Sodium sulphite E221
How used: preservative used in wine-making and other processed foods.
What you need to know: Sulphites have been associated with triggering asthma attacks. Most asthmatics are sensitive to sulphites in food.

Stannous chloride (tin) E512
How used: Antioxidant and colour-retention agent in canned and bottled foods, fruit juices.
What you need to know: Acute poisoning has been reported from ingestion of fruit juices containing concentrations of tin greater than 250mg/l – causing nausea, vomiting, diarrhoea and headaches.

Sulphur dioxide E220
How used: Very widely used preservative.
What you need to know: Sulphur dioxide reacts with a wide range of substances found in food, including various essential vitamins, minerals, enzymes and essential fats. The most common adverse reaction to sulphites is bronchial problems, particularly in those prone to asthma. Other adverse reactions may include hypotension (low blood pressure), flushing, tingling sensations and anaphylactic shock. The ILO says you should avoid E220 if you suffer from conjunctivitis, bronchitis, emphysema, bronchial asthma or cardiovascular disease.

Sunset yellow FCF, Orange/yellow S E110
How used: Widely used food colouring.
What you need to know: Some animal studies have indicated growth retardation and severe weight loss. People with asthma, rhinitis or urticaria should avoid this product.

Tartrazine	E102

How used: Widely used yellow food colour.

What you need to know: May cause allergic reactions in perhaps 15 per cent of the population. It may be a cause of asthmatic attacks and has been implicated in bouts of hyperactivity disorder in children. Those who suffer from asthma, rhinitis and urticaria may find symptoms worsen after consumption.

Source: P. Cox and P. Brusseau, Secret Ingredients *(Bantam, 1997), with permission of Peter Cox and Bantam Books*

See Chapter 23 for more details of what to look for on labels.

Go for organic

The presence of pesticide residue, particularly on fruits and vegetables, is a widely acknowledged fact. Again, it's difficult to say how significant the impact on your child's health might be. But since any toxic substance will affect all parts of the body, including the brain to some extent, it seems wise to try to avoid pesticides as much as possible.

The best way to do this is to give organic produce to your child whenever you can. And of course, organic food also contains higher amounts of health-giving nutrients. Some organic food is much more expensive than conventionally grown food, but in some cases there is little difference in price, so do what you can within your budget. Most organic food hasn't been forced to grow fast, and consequently has less water and more 'dry weight' in it. So three organic carrots would fill you up as much as four regular supermarket carrots. It's value for money: even if the price is 25 per cent more, you're getting just as much carrot at the end of the day, plus all the extra nutrients and no pesticide or herbicide residues.

But is it better to eat organic apples flown all the way from New Zealand or conventionally grown English apples that have not travelled so far? Quite a conundrum! By buying fruits and vegetables which are in season, you are more likely to able to get food that is both local and organic. That means apples and pears in winter, blackberries and plums in summer, for example. Also, go for whole lettuces rather than 'bagged' salads since these are less likely to be chemically treated to maintain 'freshness'.

Organic means much more than 'pesticide free'. Organic meat or fish has to adhere to strict rules, not only about the feed, but also about how animals are reared and the use of any growth hormones or antibiotics. It's well worth paying the extra for organic meat, eggs, farmed fish or milk.

To help prevent your child being exposed to additives, do the following.

- **Avoid foods containing chemical food additives.**

- **Be vigilant when buying food and drink.**

- **Stick to whole, natural foods as much as possible, since these should be additive-free. You will still need to check the label.**

- **Choose organic food, including meat, eggs, milk, fish, and fruit and vegetables.**

CHAPTER 9

Protecting Your Child from Brain Allergies

 As many as one in five adults and children,[66–67] and probably one in three with behavioural problems, are sensitive or have allergic reactions to common foods such as milk, wheat, yeast and eggs. Yet the knowledge that allergy to foods and chemicals can adversely affect moods and behaviour in children has been widespread, and ignored, for a very long time.

Back in the 1980s, researchers found that allergies can affect any system of the body, including the central nervous system – a result confirmed by recent double-blind controlled trials Allergies can cause a diverse range of symptoms, from fatigue, slowed thought processes, irritability and agitation, to aggressive behaviour, nervousness, anxiety, depression, ADHD, autism, hyperactivity and learning disabilities.[68–75]

Five-year-old Veronica is a case in point. She had been diagnosed with mild autism and had also been suffering her entire life with chronic constipation and regular tummy aches. When her parents brought her to us at the Brain Bio Centre, an IgG food allergy test identified an allergy to gluten. When this was removed from her diet, her parents were pleased to report a major improvement in her sociability and much improved digestion with regular bowel movements and no tummy aches.

In susceptible children, these types of symptoms can be caused by a variety of substances, though many have reactions to common foods and/or food additives. Some children, particularly those with hyperactivity or ADHD, may also react to salicylates – a natural component in many otherwise healthy foods. This will be covered in more detail in Chapter 16.

The most convincing evidence for the wide-ranging effects of food allergies comes from a well-conducted double-blind, placebo-controlled crossover trial by Dr Joseph Egger and his team, who studied 76 hyperactive children to find out whether diet can contribute to behavioural disorders. The results showed that 79 per cent of the children tested reacted adversely to artificial food colourings and preservatives, primarily tartrazine and benzoic acid, which produced a marked deterioration in behaviour.

However, Egger found that no child reacted to these alone. In fact, 48 different foods were found to produce symptoms among the children tested. For example, 64 per cent reacted to cow's milk, 59 per cent to chocolate, 49 per cent to wheat, 45 per cent to oranges, 39 per cent to eggs, 32 per cent to peanuts and 16 per cent to sugar. Interestingly, it was not only the children's behaviour that improved after their diets were modified. Most of the associated symptoms also lessened considerably, including headaches, fits, abdominal discomfort, chronic rhinitis, aches in limbs, skin rashes and mouth ulcers.[76] Other studies have reported very similar results.[77]

These studies are prime examples of how problems created by allergies often produce a multitude of physical and mental symptoms and affect many body systems. Furthermore, allergies are very specific to the individual, as are the symptoms they create.

Allergy, intolerance or sensitivity?

These days, people use the terms food allergies, food intolerances and food sensitivities almost interchangeably. So what is the difference?

The classic definition of an allergy is simply an exaggerated physical reaction to a substance where the immune system is clearly involved. The immune system, which is the body's defence system, has the ability to produce 'markers' for substances it doesn't like, the classic example being an antibody called IgE (immunoglobulin type E). When food containing the allergen is digested, it enters the bloodstream and meets its IgE marker, triggering the release of chemicals (see the figure below). These include histamine, which causes the classic symptoms of allergy – skin rashes, hayfever, rhinitis, sinusitis, asthma, eczema and anaphylaxis (a reaction where throat and mouth swell and severe asthma comes on, sometimes accompanied by a rash, rapid dropping of blood pressure, an irregular heartbeat and loss of consciousness).

All of these 'IgE-mediated' reactions are immediate and severe, and may be life-threatening. If your child has this type

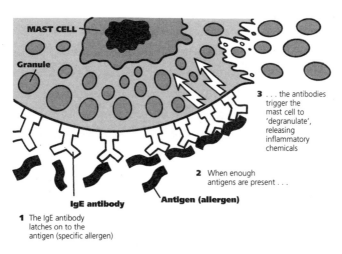

How IgE antibodies cause allergic reactions

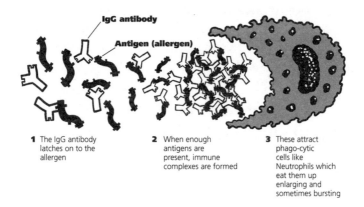

1 The IgG antibody latches on to the allergen

2 When enough antigens are present, immune complexes are formed

3 These attract phago-cytic cells like Neutrophils which eat them up enlarging and sometimes bursting

How IgG antibodies cause allergic reactions

of allergy, you probably already know about it and are keeping your child well away from the offending food.

The most common type of food allergy, however, involves a different marker – IgG. IgG allergies are often called 'delayed-onset', because the reactions may take anywhere from an hour to three days to show themselves. They are also usually far less dramatic, so they may just manifest as an uncomfortable feeling with no obvious cause. Add to this the fact that IgG reactions are often to widely consumed foods, and your child may well end up eating foods they're allergic to on a regular basis.

Food intolerances and sensitivities are reactions to food where there is no measurable antibody response. Examples of these include lactose intolerance, where a child lacks the enzyme to digest milk sugar or lactose and can develop diarrhoea and abdominal discomfort when they drink milk; or intolerance to the flavour enhancer MSG, which makes some kids hyperactive.

The top ten allergens

Any food can cause an allergic reaction but the most common include wheat and other gluten grains, milk, eggs, yeast-containing foods, shellfish, nuts, peanuts, garlic and soya. Most food allergies are a reaction to the protein in a particular food – particularly the foods we eat most frequently.

Wheat is most likely top of this list because it contains a substance called gliadin, which irritates the gut wall. Gliadin is a type of gluten, a sticky protein that allows pockets of air to form when combined with yeast – hence allowing bread dough to rise. Eating a lot of wheat products isn't good for anyone, and especially not for your child if they have developed an allergy. The connections between wheat allergy, autism and ADHD are well established (see Chapters 16 and 17).

Rye, barley and oats contain much less gluten as well as different kinds of it. So if your child is allergic to wheat, they may be able to tolerate rye, barley and oats; while some children who are allergic to wheat, rye and barley can tolerate oats, which contains no gliadin.

Dairy products, including cheese and yoghurt, cause allergic reactions in many children. Some children can seemingly tolerate goat's or sheep's milk, but not cow's milk. However, this is more likely due to their consuming less dairy overall: goat's and sheep's milk and cheese tend to come in much smaller cartons and blocks and are not universally available, after all. Allergic reactions often include a blocked nose, frequent colds, bloating and indigestion, 'thick' head, fatigue, earaches and headaches.

Getting to grips with allergies

Of all the avenues so far researched, the link between behavioural problems and allergy is the best established. If your child is hyperactive or prone to unexplained mood swings, allergy testing is likely to be worthwhile. Let's take a look at the options.

Allergy tests

If your child has a history of infantile colic, eczema, asthma, ear infections, hayfever, seasonal allergies, digestive problems (including bloating, constipation and diarrhoea), frequent colds and any behavioural or learning problems, you should suspect a delayed food allergy and should have him or her tested to identify the culprit. The best test is IgG ELISA, which uses a finger-prick blood sample taken at home with a home test kit.

Testing is best done under the guidance of a nutritional therapist or allergy expert, who can devise a diet for your child that cuts out all allergy-provoking foods and includes suitable alternatives. See Resources, page 278, for details on how to arrange allergy testing, and how to find a nutritional therapist in your area.

An alternative method of identifying food allergies is an elimination and challenge diet. This involves removing any likely culprits from your child's diet for a period of time (often from two weeks to three months) and noting any changes in behaviour and mental and physical symptoms. Then the foods can be reintroduced in a controlled way while simultaneously monitoring your child's state of health. It has to be said, however, that this method has many shortcomings because the range of foods a child can react to is so broad.

As you'll know if you or your child has an IgE allergy, the food in question (such as peanuts or shrimp) will have to be avoided for life. But IgG allergies – which have a relatively gentle, delayed effect – may not be long-term. By identifying the foods that your child is allergic to, strictly avoiding them for around six months and improving digestive health, your child may lose their allergy to them. But in some cases, an IgG allergy reaction is, like IgE allergies, for life. (If you'd like to find out more, read *Hidden Food Allergies* by Patrick Holford and Dr James Braly.)

The gut factor

Digestive problems are often the underlying factor in a delayed-onset, or IgG, food allergy. Many children have excessively 'leaky' digestive tracts, which means that partially undigested proteins enter their bloodstream and trigger a reaction.

The leakiness can develop with frequent use of antibiotics or aspirin, gastrointestinal infection, a yeast infestation such as candidiasis, or a deficiency in essential fats, vitamin A or zinc. So identifying and avoiding what your child is reacting to is just half the equation with an IgG food allergy. The other half is getting their digestion back into gear (see page 177 for more on this).

A child who has food allergy symptoms such as frequent ear or chest infections is likely to be prescribed antibiotics by their doctor. This can make the gut leakier and worsen the allergy, leading in turn to more antibiotics in a vicious round of unnecessary ill health. Clearly, it's best to deal with the root cause of the symptoms by identifying food allergens and removing them from your child's diet rather than relying on antibiotics for short-term relief and long-term worsening of the problem.

There are a number of ways to test for, and reduce, your child's allergic potential.

- **Take wheat and dairy products out of their diet strictly for one month or more and see how they feel. In any case, try to limit these food groups in your child's diet by not having them every day.**

- **Improve your child's digestion by including plenty of fresh fruit, vegetables, seeds and fish in their diet, which contain essential fats and zinc.**

- Keep antibiotics to a minimum – they damage the digestive tract.

- If you suspect your child has a food allergy, have an IgG ELISA food allergy test and see a clinical nutritional therapist. They can both test what your child is allergic to, devise a course of action to reduce their allergic potential and ensure that your child's diet remains balanced and healthy while excluding these problem foods.

PART 2

Give Your Child a Head Start

We were all taught how the right foods will give us strong bones and healthy physiques. But recent research has looked beyond the strictly physical into the realm of mind. Eating the best foods has been proven to boost IQ, improve mood and behaviour, hone memory and concentration, and sharpen reading and writing skills. In this part of the book you'll discover how to maximise your child's potential for better school performance while helping them to enjoy life and feel personally fulfilled.

CHAPTER 10

Testing, Testing

Are your child's mind and memory sharp? Can they concentrate and stay alert for an hour? Is their mood stable? Do they sleep well, get to sleep easily, and wake up fizzing with energy and raring to go? Or are they often exhausted, easily distracted, and prone to overreact, or get upset or angry easily?

Now you've learnt the basics about the nutrients your child needs for optimum nutrition it's time to go close up on what your child's intelligence is all about.

First, we are all different due to our genes, and your child will inherit their own unique strengths and weaknesses. But genes are less important than you might think – they are only part of the story when it comes to how your child develops. These bits of DNA are really just the instructions inside each cell to build proteins out of the amino acids that you eat. So we inherit slightly different abilities to build certain proteins, and that in turn changes not only how we look, but also how we think. That's because proteins make enzymes and enzymes make the neurotransmitters that are so key to how we think and feel. Since proteins, enzymes and neurotransmitters are all made from nutrients, it's no surprise to find that food directly affects the brain.

The facets of intelligence

As we discussed in Chapter 3, there are three kinds of intelligence: intellectual, emotional and physical.

Intellectual intelligence we are well aware of. It concerns your child's ability to learn, remember, solve problems, think laterally, concentrate and so on.

Emotional intelligence we can define as the ability to monitor one's own and others' emotions and react appropriately, channel our emotions to serve a goal, respond with empathy, and maintain healthy relationships. Being sensitive to how another child feels and saying a kind word, not overreacting when things aren't going their own way, or being able to say how they feel are all part of your child's emotional intelligence.

Physical intelligence involves overall physical fitness, balance, agility and coordination, anticipation, reaction time, strength and flexibility. Not bumping into things and hurting yourself on a daily basis, or being able to learn a physical skill, are examples of physical intelligence.

All these kinds of intelligence involve the brain, yet psychological and social theories of intelligence and behaviour often seem to glance over this fundamental fact. Put simply, if your child's brain isn't working properly, they can't think straight or feel balanced. Most of the problems we humans create in our own and the larger world come about when we don't think clearly, and then respond with inappropriate emotional reactions. To look at it another way, whatever your archetype of an 'enlightened' person might be – whether Buddha or Christ, Gandhi or the Dalai Lama, Einstein or Edison – the chances are that you define their enlightenment as clear thinking and responses that aren't at the mercy of every passing emotion.

But are such qualities something we are born with, or are they acquired? And do they depend in any way on nutrition?

Even though there's obviously an inherited aspect to intelligence, we are going to show you how optimum nutrition promotes all-round intelligence by nourishing your child's brain.

Before doing so, here's a simple checklist of questions to help you gauge your child's current mental, emotional and physical state. Given that age is going to determine ability, please answer these questions, where appropriate, in relation to other children's ability at the same age, or to their peers at school.

Your Child's Brain Check

Concentration and focus

- [ ] Is your child often restless and overactive?
- [ ] Does your child disturb other people?
- [ ] Does your child fail to finish things?
- [ ] Does your child constantly fidget or squirm when they're meant to be still?
- [ ] Is your child inattentive or easily disturbed?
- [ ] Does your child get dizzy or irritable if they don't eat often?

IQ, memory and creative thinking

- [ ] Would you describe your child as a slow learner?
- [ ] Do they lose the plot in films or stories?
- [ ] Do they find it hard to do calculations in their head? (age 6 plus)
- [ ] Do they find it hard to make up imaginary stories?
- [ ] Would you describe your child as forgetful?
- [ ] Is your child able to entertain themselves if left alone?

Reading and writing

- [ ] Is your child behind at school with his/her reading?
- [ ] Is your child behind at school in his/her writing?
- [ ] If you ask them, does your child say that the words move on the page?

☐ Is their spelling particularly bad or do they get the letters in the wrong place?

☐ Do they frequently get their 'left' and 'right' confused?

☐ Has your child been suspected or confirmed as dyslexic?

Mood and behaviour

☐ Is your child especially excitable and impulsive?

☐ Do they expect their demands to be immediately met?

☐ Do they become easily frustrated?

☐ Are they prone to outbursts of temper or temper tantrums?

☐ Does your child's mood change quickly and are they often unhappy?

☐ Does your child cry easily and often?

Physical coordination

☐ Would you describe your child as clumsy?

☐ Does your child frequently have cuts and bruises and bump into things?

☐ Are they incompetent with ball sports?

☐ Are they slow to learn physical activities?

☐ Can they throw a ball 3 feet in the air, clap, and catch it? (age 6 plus)

☐ Do they have difficulty in balancing activities?

If your child scores three or more 'yes' answers in any of these sections, or has a total score over 10 (the maximum score is 25), then it's very likely that following our recommendations will help your child think and feel better.

The following four chapters explain what steps you can take to optimise your child's potential.

CHAPTER 11

Thinking Faster, Boosting IQ

 It may surprise you to know that you can boost your child's intelligence quotient or IQ score at any age. Some people argue that your real 'intelligence' – how smart you are – is innate, something you're born with. But the truth is that your ability to make intelligent decisions depends not only on this aspect of intelligence, but also on the clarity of your mind, how quickly you can think, your attention, how long you can concentrate and how good your memory is. All of these can be improved with optimum nutrition.

Twelve-year-old Rachel is a case in point. She had been diagnosed with Global Developmental Delay at four years of age and before coming to us at the Brain Bio Centre, her IQ was measured at 45 points. We assessed her nutrient status and found that she was low in many key brain nutrients including zinc, magnesium and the B vitamins. Her diet simply did not contain the nutrients that she needed. Improvements in her diet such as increasing the amount of freshly prepared food that she ate and taking a high-dose multivitamin and mineral formula along with some fish oils resulted in a 25 point increase in her IQ after ten months.

This should not be surprising. In Part 1 of this book we saw how the brain, composed of a highly complex network of neurons, is made from what we eat. Thinking is a pattern of activity across this network. The messengers relaying the thoughts are neurotransmitters, which again are made from and directly affected by what we eat. When we learn, we actually change the wiring of the brain. When we think, we change the activity of neurotransmitters.

So we and our children shape the way we think, to a huge degree. This was the logic that made us investigate, in 1986, whether giving a child an optimal intake of nutrients used by the brain and nervous system would improve intellectual performance.

Feeding the intellect

Intellectual performance is generally measured as IQ, with a score of 100 considered to be average for whatever age of the child being tested. About 5 per cent of children score above 125, and less than 10 per cent score below 80, which is considered to be educationally subnormal and in need of special help.

Way back in 1960 there was evidence of a link between IQ and nutrition. A study by Dr Albert Kubala and colleagues in the US had shown that higher levels of vitamin C were associated with an increased IQ. Kubala divided 351 students into high and low vitamin C groups, depending on levels of the vitamin in their blood. The students' IQ was then measured and found to average 113 and 109 respectively: those with higher blood levels of the vitamin had IQs averaging 4.5 points higher.[78]

Then, in 1981, another researcher looked at the effect of multivitamins on children with mental retardation. Having heard that some children with Down's syndrome had made big increases in IQ by taking multivitamins, Dr Ruth Harrell ran the first ever 'double-blind' trial, giving 22 mentally retarded children high-strength multivitamin and mineral supplements, or placebos.[79] After four months the IQs of the children taking the supplements had improved by between 5 and 10 points, while those on the placebo had shown no change. All the children were then put on the supplements and, after a further four months, the average IQ improvement was 10.2 points.

But up to then, no one had tested the effects of vitamins on normal children at school. So in 1986 we decided to see whether giving a high-potency multivitamin would improve the IQ of ordinary schoolchildren.

Working with Gwillym Roberts, a headmaster and nutritional therapist who had trained at the Institute for Optimum Nutrition, we worked out what combination of nutrients would optimally nourish the brain. Roberts then gave these to a pilot group of students at his school, measuring their IQ before and after. Their non-verbal IQ went up by a staggering ten points. (Non-verbal IQ, which involves activities such as shape pattern-matching, is considered more innate than verbal IQ, which varies more according to the testee's grasp of English and schooling.)

To test this further, Roberts devised a randomised, double-blind, placebo-controlled trial with David Benton, professor of psychology at Swansea University. Once again, after eight months on the supplements, the non-verbal IQs in those taking the supplements had risen by an average of over 10 points.[80]

This now famous IQ study, published in the *Lancet*, spawned more than a dozen similar studies to test the idea further. The next big one, conducted by professors Stephen Schoenthaler, John Yudkin, world-famous psychologist Hans Eysenck and Dr Linus Pauling, involved 615 children given much lower levels of nutrients, at RDA levels. Once again, the results showed that the simple addition of a vitamin and mineral supplement could increase IQ scores by as much as 20 points, with an average increase of at least 4.5 points, this time over three months.[81]

The truth is that a 4.5 IQ point shift would get many thousands of educationally subnormal children reclassified and returned to mainstream schools. More comprehensive nutritional programmes have brought even children with IQs in the 40s back into the normal range. But your child doesn't have to be in this category to benefit. Children with high IQs have also shown improvement.

The results of our earlier trials have been replicated more than a dozen times and shown to work in 10 out of 13 well-designed trials.[82] (A study at Kings College London,[83] which at one month was too short, showed no effect.) You do, however, 'need' to be sub-optimally nourished. In other words, once you're getting your ideal intake of nutrients, more won't make you even brighter.

The consistent, positive benefit of giving your child supplements is also likely to last for life, according to a recent survey carried out by Aberdeen University's Department of Mental Health, which found that supplement use also correlates with higher IQ scores later in life. This survey also emphasised the link between getting enough omega-3 fats and sharp intelligence.[84]

How nutrients boost IQ

But how exactly do nutrients increase IQ scores? Wendy Snowden, a researcher from Reading University's psychology department, decided to investigate. Once again, schoolchildren were given supplements or a placebo.[85] After 10 weeks, the children taking supplements showed significant increases in non-verbal IQ scores, but not in verbal IQ scores. A close analysis of performance in the IQ tests showed the same error rate, but the children were able to work faster and attempt more questions after the 10 weeks of supplementation. For the verbal IQ test, all children completed all questions, so there was no room for improvement in work rate.

All this suggests that vitamin and mineral supplements effectively increase the speed of information processing in the brain – clearly a significant factor in IQ and, by implication, in intelligence. These amazing nutrients seem to help children think faster, and also concentrate for longer – which we'll explore in more detail in the next chapter.

Go-faster food

Certain vitamins, minerals and fats seem particularly good at boosting brain speed. Let's look at them now.

Brain-accelerating vitamins and minerals

When it comes to fast cognition, there is good reason to 'think zinc'. A recent trial involving 209 children aged 10 to 11 in North Dakota showed remarkable results in how zinc supplements help speed up thinking.[86] The children were given a juice drink containing either 10mg of zinc, 20mg of zinc or none. The RDA for zinc for this age group is 10mg, so it's likely that these children would have been getting something like this level of the mineral.

At the beginning and end of the study, students had to perform a number of tests designed to measure mental skills, like attention, memory, problem-solving and hand-to-eye coordination.

Examples include tapping a key on the keyboard as fast as possible, using a mouse to follow an object moving across the screen, searching a group of objects for two of a kind, learning and remembering lists of words or simple geometric patterns, and categorising objects.

Compared to the students who received no additional zinc, students given 20mg zinc each day decreased reaction time on a visual memory test by 12 per cent, versus 6 per cent; increased correct answers on a word recognition test by 9 per cent, versus 3 per cent; and increased scores on a test requiring sustained attention and vigilance by 6 per cent, versus 1 per cent.

This illustrates why the RDA level of nutrients, which is the amount needed to keep your child from developing a deficiency disease (such as scurvy, from a lack of vitamin C), are hopelessly inadequate if you want to keep your child's brain optimally nourished. Other nutrients that boost IQ beyond RDA levels include vitamin B1, B6, B12, and folic acid. Studies with teenagers, for example, have found that 50mg of vitamin B1 a day improves speed of thinking[87] – yet the RDA is a mere 1.4mg!

So how much is enough? The RDA issue points to the need to know how much of the important vitamins and minerals your child needs to take to accelerate their thinking. Some die-hard dieticians still believe the mantra that your child 'can get all the nutrients they need from a well-balanced diet'. While we encourage you wholeheartedly to feed your child a well-balanced diet, as defined in Part 1, the evidence in dozens of studies reported in this book shows that achieving more than the basic RDA levels of nutrients will boost intelligence. And our original study back in the mid-1980s, where children were given the highest levels of vitamins and minerals, produced the biggest increase in IQ scores.

The chart below shows the levels of vitamins and minerals that we recommend you give your child every day, assuming you also ensure their diet is the best possible too.

The easiest way to give your child all these vitamins and minerals is via a daily multi. The trouble with most multivitamin/minerals combinations is there aren't many good-tasting, chewable types that pack in these levels of nutrients. We've searched high and low and list the ones worth buying in the Resources section on page 280, including supplements that dissolve in water. Of the chewable supplements, most involve taking, for example, one chewable tablet for every two years of life. So a six year-old would take three a day.

The Ideal Daily Supplement Programme: Vitamins and Minerals

Age	Less than 1	1	2	3–4	5–6	7–8	9–11
Nutrient							
Vitamins							
A (retinol) (mcg)	500	600	700	800	1000	1500	2000
D (mcg)	1	1.25	1.5	1.75	2.25	2.5	2.5
E (mg)	13	13	17	20	23	30	40
C (mg)	100	100	200	300	400	500	600
B1 (thiamine) (mg)	5	5	6	8	12	16	20
B2 (riboflavin) (mg)	5	5	6	8	12	16	20
B3 (niacin) (mg)	7	10	14	16	18	20	22
B5 (pantothenic acid)	10	10	15	20	25	30	35
B6 (pyridoxine) (mg)	5	5	7	10	12	16	20
B12 (mcg)	5	6	7	8	9	10	10
Folic acid (mcg)	100	100	120	140	160	180	200
Biotin (mcg)	30	40	50	60	70	80	90
Minerals							
Calcium (mg)	150	160	170	180	190	200	210
Magnesium (mg)	50	60	70	80	90	100	110
Iron (mg)	4	5	6	7	8	9	10
Zinc (mg)	4	5	6	7	9	11	15
Manganese (mcg)	300	300	350	400	500	700	1000
Iodine (mcg)	50	75	100	125	150	175	200
Chromium (mcg)	15	17	20	23	25	27	30
Selenium (mcg)	10	15	20	25	28	30	35

Essential fat – oiling the mental wheels

Back in the 1980s, the extent of supplementation for children was vitamins and minerals. Today we know that supplementing omega-3 fats is just as important. They not only improve your child's emotional intelligence and behaviour, as we'll see in Chapter 14; they also keep those mental wheels well oiled and running fast and smoothly.

The levels of omega-3 fats at birth, especially DHA – the 'brain-building' fat – predict intellectual development later in life.[88-89] And there is overwhelming evidence that supplementing DHA in infants improves the speed of their thinking and other measures of mental performance at ages 3,[90] 4,[91] 6 and 8.[92] So the effects of optimum nutrition during pregnancy and early infancy are long-lasting. Although not proven yet, it is highly likely that supplementation with fish oils rich in omega-3s throughout infancy and childhood will maximise a child's intellectual development.

Eating oily coldwater fish is an excellent way of getting more omega-3s into your child's diet, and the chart below shows the amounts of DHA in each type. As we saw in Chapter 3, however, be careful with fresh tuna (go for the steaks, as the tinned variety has much less omega-3): it does tend to be high in mercury, so limit it to two or three times a month. And with salmon, stick with wild or organic farmed fish.

Best Fish for Brain Fats	
Amount of DHA in 100g (3½oz)	
Mackerel	1,400mg
Herring	1,000mg
Sardines	1,000mg
Tuna	900mg
Anchovy	900mg
Salmon	800mg
Trout	500mg

An ideal intake of DHA a day for your child is in the order of 300mg to 400mg a day. So if they are eating 100g of oily fish (preferably sardines, mackerel or herring) three times a week, they'll be doing very well. Alternatively, they can take a supplement of fish oils containing DHA. A good one can provide up to 200mg.

The best source of all, at least for babies, is breast milk. It's naturally rich in DHA, particularly if the mother is eating fish or flaxseeds. Breastfed babies not only have higher IQs 10 years down the track,[93] and better results in exams; they also have fewer mental health problems.[94]

In Chapters 15 and 16 we'll show you some of the extraordinary results already achieved in children with dyslexia, ADHD and other learning difficulties. You'll also learn how EPA, another kind of omega-3 fat rich in fish oil, seems to help these children more than DHA. Hence we recommend that you supplement both DHA and EPA.

Age	Less than 1	1	2	3–4	5–6	7–8	9–11
The Ideal Daily Supplement Programme: Omega-3s							
Essential fats							
EPA (mg)	100	150	200	250	300	350	400
DHA (mg)	100	125	150	175	200	225	250

Fish oils are the best way of supplementing omega-3s, but they're not to everyone's liking. However, nowadays there are many supplements, gels, oils and capsules cleverly flavoured to entice your child into developing the vital habit of supplementing fish oils every day.

Because oily fish can contain mercury, as we've pointed out, the fish oil supplements you give your child should be purified to be mercury free. All those we list in Resources are not only free from mercury, but also come out best of those tested for PCBs and other pollutants now sadly endemic in our seas.

So the first steps to maximising your child's IQ are the following.

- Ensure an optimum intake of vitamins and minerals, both from diet and supplements, by giving your child a high-strength children's multivitamin and mineral supplement every day, not one based solely on the RDAs. For specific supplement recommendations, see Chapter 26.

- Optimise your child's intake of essential fats, especially omega-3 fats, by giving them flaxseeds, oily fish and/or fish oil supplements every day.

These are the basics. But there's still plenty more that you can do to enhance your child's all-round intelligence, coming up in the next three chapters.

CHAPTER 12

Developing Concentration and a Sharp Memory

 As a parent, you'll have seen at least one child who can't sit still, fidgets all the time and seems to lack a normal attention span. In fact, 'attention deficit' has become one of the most common problems afflicting today's children. Being able to stay focused on a task, project or piece of schoolwork is a key part of maximising a child's abilities. As we saw in the last chapter, achieving optimum nutrition through diet and supplements raises IQ partly because children concentrate better. Vitamins, however, aren't the key factor for concentration. It's sugar – or more precisely, blood sugar balance.

Key to concentration – blood sugar balance

As we saw in Chapter 2, keeping an even blood sugar level is critical to intelligence because it's this, more than anything else, that affects your child's ability to concentrate over long periods of time.

Why so? In a nutshell, it's all down to the brain's fuel, glucose – the sugar derived from the carbohydrates we eat. If over time your child eats too much of the wrong kind of carbohydrates, such as sweets and refined starchy foods, their blood and brain sugar levels start rollercoasting. When their blood sugar suddenly dips, their concentration can wander, and any aggressive behaviour can get worse.[95–99]

This is why it is absolutely vital that your child eats a healthy breakfast and doesn't snack on sugary foods and drinks. A recent school survey found that almost two-thirds (65 per cent) of pupils eat sweets, chocolate bars or biscuits at least once a day; 64 per cent drink fizzy drinks or squashes that contain sugar; and 31 per cent eat chips or other fried potato snacks and crisps. All of these give your child a rush of sugar to their brain, followed abruptly by a sugar crash and poor concentration.

Aptos Middle School in San Francisco, California, took this message to heart and removed all sugared soft drinks from its vending machines. They also banned all refined carbohydrate snacks and foods, such as French fries, from the cafeteria. Since the nutrition changes were put into place, administrators and teachers report better student behaviour after lunch, fewer afternoon visits to the counselling office, less litter in the schoolyard, and more students sitting down to eat. The school also reported higher scores on standardised tests. Their motto now? 'No empty calories!'

Queensbury School in Dunstable, Bedfordshire, may be the first British school to follow suit. The school recently removed all fizzy drinks, crisps and sweets from its vending machines and started to provide free drinking water. Nigel Hill, the head-teacher, said: 'We took the ethical decision that is facing thousands of schools. Do you put students' health first, or the money you can make from selling them chocolate and fizzy drinks?' One year on, deputy head Karen Hayward, who is in charge of the project, told us that removing the vending machine selling fizzy drinks was literally the best decision the school had ever made. There has been a definite improvement, especially in pupils with ADHD-type problems.

The importance of eating breakfast

Other schools have set up 'breakfast clubs' to encourage children who don't eat breakfast at home to get into the habit of having it. If that sounds peculiar to you – because your kids always leave the house set up by a plate of eggs or a bowl of porridge – you should know that a third of children in Britain don't have a proper breakfast. But those who do have much better concentration and attention spans, according to a number of studies.[100]

Breakfast should become a golden rule in any household, but what reaches the table needs some thought. For instance, school breakfast clubs are a great idea – but some reportedly serve crisps, doughnuts and other junk food, so if your child attends one it's vital to check and see what they're serving.

The best breakfast is a low-GL one. As we saw in Chapter 2, low-GL carbohydrates are the kind that keep your child's blood sugar even. Cereal is an easy and deservedly popular breakfast choice, but one with a number of pitfalls – few commercial cereals are low-GL. Let's look at the options in the chart below.

Glycaemic Load of Breakfast Cereals			
Food	Serve size (g)	Looks like	GLs per serving
Low-carb muesli (see *The Holford Low-GL Diet Cookbook*)	60	Large bowl	4
Porridge made from rolled oats	30	Large bowl	2
GoodCarb Original Granola	50	Medium bowl	5
Get Up & Go	30		3
Get Up & Go with strawberries and 1/2 pint of milk (E)	30	1/2 pint drink	8.5
All-Bran™	30	1 small serving	6
Muesli, gluten-free	30	1 medium serving	7
Muesli (Alpen)	30	1 serving	10
Muesli, Natural	30	1 serving	10

Food	Serve size (g)	Looks like	GLs per serving
Raisin Bran™ (Kellogg's)	30	1 medium serving	12
Weetabix™	25	2 biscuits	11
Bran Flakes™	30	1 medium serving	13
Sultana Bran™ (Kellogg's)	30	1 medium serving	14
Special K™ (Kellogg's)	30	1 medium serving	14
Shredded Wheat™	40	2 biscuits	20
Cheerios™	30	1 medium serving	15
Frosties™ (Kellogg's)	30	1 medium serving	15
Grapenuts™	30	1 medium serving	15
Golden Wheats™ (Kellogg's)	30	1 medium serving	16
Puffed Wheat	30	1 medium serving	16
Honey Smacks™ (Kellogg's)	30	1 medium serving	16
Cornflakes, Crunchy Nut™ (Kellogg's)	30	1 medium serving	17
Coco Pops™	30	1 medium serving	20
Rice Krispies™ (Kellogg's)	30	1 medium serving	21
Cornflakes™ (Kellogg's)	30	1 medium serving	21

The goal is for breakfast to be no more than 10 GLs, including added fruit – a score somewhat depending on your child's age and size. So ideally, the cereal part should be no more than 5 GLs. As you can see, that rules out almost every branded cereal.

The Consumers' Association checked out 28 branded cereals, and found that nine contained 40 per cent sugar or more! The worst options included Quaker Sugar Puffs™, which contained 49g per 100g, and Frosties™. A bowl of Frosties™ contained the equivalent of four heaped teaspoons of sugar. There are many different names for added sugar to check for on the label. These include sugar, fructose, glucose, malt, honey, inverted glucose syrup and dextrose, to name just a few. From the point of view of sugar content, the best packaged cereal was Weetabix ReadyBrek™ (original).

The best breakfast cereal option by far is porridge oat flakes, which can be eaten hot and cooked or cold and raw, sweetened with fresh fruit. GoodCarb Original Granola is also excellent, as is Low GL Get Up and Go, a breakfast shake powder that you blend with milk and berries (see Resources, page 282, for suppliers). Alternatively, you could make your own low-GL muesli with oats, seeds, nuts and oat bran, and sweeten your child's daily portion with fresh fruit.

But you don't have to give your child cereal. Ring the changes with high-protein, low-GL and thoroughly delectable options such as eggs or kippers, either served with wholegrain toast. (See Chapter 24 for other practical and delicious breakfasts.)

Grazing the low-GL way

Eating low-GL, slow-releasing carbohydrates and grazing, not gorging, is the best way to avoid blood sugar dips. So it's good to encourage healthy snacking from the start by having a bountiful bowl of fruit available at all times. The best fruits are apples, pears, peaches, and any berries, from strawberries to blueberries. Provided your child is not too young to be nibbling on nuts or seeds, a handful of pumpkin seeds, sunflower seeds or almonds is also a great snack. As far as school is concerned, you can always send your child to school armed with an apple and a tub of nuts and seeds.

Other good snacks are oat cakes. Choose rough oat cakes that are sugar-free, such as Nairn's, because these have the lowest GL score. They also make oat biscuits which, although they do contain sugar, contain a fraction of that found in other biscuits; so they're good as a treat. It's also an excellent idea to have a non-sugary spread, such as peanut or any other nut butter, in your store cupboard. A teaspoon spread on an oat cake makes for a delicious, sustaining and healthy snack.

Farewell to the fizz

The worst offenders, as far as sugar is concerned, are sweet, fizzy drinks. A 2-litre bottle of cola contains more than 40 teaspoons of sugar! Most of this category of drinks are best avoided. The best to encourage is water: if a child is brought up drinking water when thirsty, that is what they'll drink. Of all the fruit juices, apple, pear and orange are best, but make sure you pick 100 per cent fresh fruit juices, dilute at least half and half with water, and don't make it a staple. Avoid products called 'fruit juice drinks': these inevitably contain added sugar.

Natural memory boosters

Concentration is one thing, but once your child has finished a task, what about their recall of it? Memory is vital in school and beyond. Let's look at which nutrients are key in this context.

Phosphatidyl choline

The main brain chemical involved in memory is acetylcholine. As we saw in Chapter 4, this is derived from phosphatidyl choline, a phospholipid in foods.

The richest dietary sources of phosphatidyl choline are egg yolks and fish, especially sardines. A child needs about 500mg to 1,000mg of phosphatidyl choline a day to maximise mental function. Most lecithin contains about 20 per cent phosphatidyl choline, so your child would need 2.5 to 5g of lecithin a day. You can also buy 'Hi–PC' lecithin, which is twice as rich in phosphatidyl choline, so you would only need 1 to 2.5g day, or a level teaspoon.

However, choline isn't the only substance you need to make more acetylcholine. Vitamin B5 (pantothenic acid) is essential for the formation of acetylcholine in the body, as are vitamins B1, B12 and also vitamin C. So memories are also made of a good multi.

In Chapter 4 we saw how recent research reveals that taking choline during pregnancy can result in offspring with 'super-brains'.[101] But supplementing choline later on helps children and adults alike. Dr Ladd and colleagues at the West Valley College in Saratoga, California, gave 80 students a single 25g dose of phosphatidyl choline, and found a significant improvement in memory 90 minutes later, most likely due to the improved responses of slow learners.[102] If you combine choline with other 'smart' nutrients such as pyroglutamate (see page 124), you can achieve the same memory-boosting effect at lower amounts.

Phosphatidyl serine

Phosphatidyl serine or PS – which like PC is found in eggs and organ meats – is another phospholipid essential to memory. Along with essential fats and protein, PS is one of the main building materials in the 'docking ports' on neurons – the receptor sites where neurotransmitters latch on to deliver their messages. As such, PS is very important to the smooth working of your child's brain.

DMAE

DMAE (again, sardines are a rich source) is a precursor of choline that crosses much more easily from the blood into brain cells, accelerating the brain's production of acetylcholine. It reduces anxiety, stops the mind racing, improves concentration, promotes learning and acts as a mild brain stimulant.

Slight chemical variations of DMAE have been marketed as the drug Deaner or Deanol, which have proven highly effective in numerous double-blind trials in helping children with learning problems, ADHD, memory and behaviour problems. In one survey by Dr Bernard Rimland in California, Deaner was found to be almost twice as effective in treating children with ADHD as the drug Ritalin, and without the side-effects.[103]

The ideal dose for memory enhancement is 100mg for children under seven, up to 500mg for teenagers, taken in the morning or midday, not last thing in the evening. (Too much can overstimulate, and is therefore not recommended for people diagnosed with schizophrenia, mania or epilepsy.) Don't expect immediate results. DMAE can take two to three weeks to work, but it's worth waiting for.

Glutamine and pyroglutamate – amazing brain fuel

While acetylcholine is the major player as far as memory is concerned, many neurotransmitters are also involved. Some stimulate mental processes, while others prevent information overload. A good balance works best.

For example, the stimulating neurotransmitter GABA, which is made from the amino acid glutamine, helps forge links between memories and calms down an overexcited nervous system. However, a slight variation in this key memory molecule, called glutamate, can literally overexcite neurons to death if there is too much of it 'free' or unbound in the bloodstream. (This is how MSG or monosodium glutamate turns up the volume on tastes, but can be a bad thing in large quantities.) Another form of this amino acid, pyroglutamate, greatly enhances learning. Pyroglutamate is found in many foods, including fish, dairy products, fruits and vegetables.

Here are the three ways pyroglutamate helps improve your memory and mental alertness:

- Increases acetylcholine production

- Boosts the number of receptors for acetylcholine

- Improves communication between the left and right hemispheres of the brain.

So it improves the brain's 'talking and listening', plus cooperation between the two hemispheres. As a result, learning, memory, concentration and the speed of reflexes will all benefit.

Glutamine is the most abundant amino acid in the cerebrospinal fluid surrounding the brain. It can be used directly as fuel for the brain and has been shown to enhance mood and mental performance and decrease addictive tendencies.[104] In studies designed to test whether glutamine proved safe in large doses, researchers from Boston Women's Hospital in Massachusetts gave healthy volunteers between 40 and 60g a day. Not only was it shown to be safe, but one of the side-effects was an enhanced ability to solve problems on continuous performance tests. This study was only five days long, showing that glutamine has an immediate effect, and possibly a greater effect over time.[105]

Glutamine is an important nutrient for the brain and there is good logic to adding 500mg to 1,000mg, depending on age, to your child's daily supplement programme, especially if they are having learning problems. It can be bought in powder form; some supplements contain either glutamine or pyroglutamate. As with all the other brain nutrients we've discussed in this chapter – DMAE, phospatidyl choline and serine – it's best taken in the morning as it has a stimulative effect on your child's mental function.

So there are a number of simple steps you can take to improve your child's concentration and memory.

- **Always give your child a healthy, low-GL breakfast.**

- **Encourage snacking on fruit, nuts, seeds, oat cakes or, in moderation, oat biscuits.**

- **Avoid sugary drinks, choosing water and half-and-half diluted juices instead.**

- **Add a level teaspoon of lecithin high in phosphatidyl choline to your child's cereal each morning, or a dessert-spoon of regular lecithin.**

- Alternatively, consider giving your child a supplement that contains a combination of the brain food nutrients listed above – phosphatidyl choline, phosphatidyl serine, DMAE, pyroglutamate.

CHAPTER 13

Revving Up Reading and Writing

At the age of five, some kids are just learning their letters and others are reading Hans Christian Andersen – and there are huge differences, too, in their progress with pencil and paper. All this is perfectly natural. When it comes to reading and writing, children develop at their own pace: they all take a different length of time and have a different natural aptitude for these vital skills. There can be a gender difference, too, as boys often develop later in this regard.

That said, if your child struggles with reading or writing and is behind at school, you may be able to help them by improving their nutrition.

Reece is a case in point. As he was behind at school, Reece decided he didn't like reading. He also couldn't sit still for long. His mother had taken him to a psychologist, but that hadn't helped. As part of a TV trial for London's *This Morning* programme, we encouraged Reece and his mother to carry out a one-week 'experiment'. Reece was to be given ground seeds on his cereal and more fish (for essential fats), less meat, no sugar or foods with chemical additives, and a special drink called Optio, which is the equivalent of a multivitamin and mineral in fruit juice.

Opposite, you can see an example of Reece's handwriting before the changes to his diet, and, overleaf one week after. Not only did he write one and a half pages in the same amount of time, compared to four lines before the diet, but his handwriting also improved dramatically. His mother, who was sceptical about the trial, said:

'I thought that nothing could calm this child down. He was very fidgety, he was hard to get into bed, hyperactive and constantly on the go and with occasional tantrums. Now he's a completely different child. He's a lot calmer and he wants to do more at school. In two weeks his reading has gone up a level. He doesn't get so overexcited and he's much nicer to be with. We are definitely going to stick with the diet.'

At the end of the first month Reece's reading level had gone up a year! Now he loves reading and his writing is improving in leaps and bounds.

Reading and writing problems are often due to perceptual difficulties. One of the first things to rule out is short- or long-sightedness. Often children who struggle to read and write simply have poor eyesight. Improving their eyesight with natural vision improvement methods such as the Bates Method (see Resources) can bring considerable improvement. Alternatively, get them tested for glasses. However, just as often, the problem lies not in the ability of the eyes to focus, but in the ability of the brain to process the information correctly.

An extreme example of this is dyslexia, which we cover in detail in Chapter 15. If you are concerned that your child might have dyslexia, and know that there's a history of literacy difficulties in your family, complete the Dyslexia Check below. To answer some of the questions you may need to see your child in the classroom setting, and/or consult their teacher.

✳✳✳✳✳✳✳✳✳✳✳✳✳✳✳✳✳✳✳✳✳✳✳✳✳✳✳

23.01.03
L.O. – to write a story with a moral

Activity

Write your own story in which the main character learns the
importance of saying please and thank you.

Reece's handwriting before

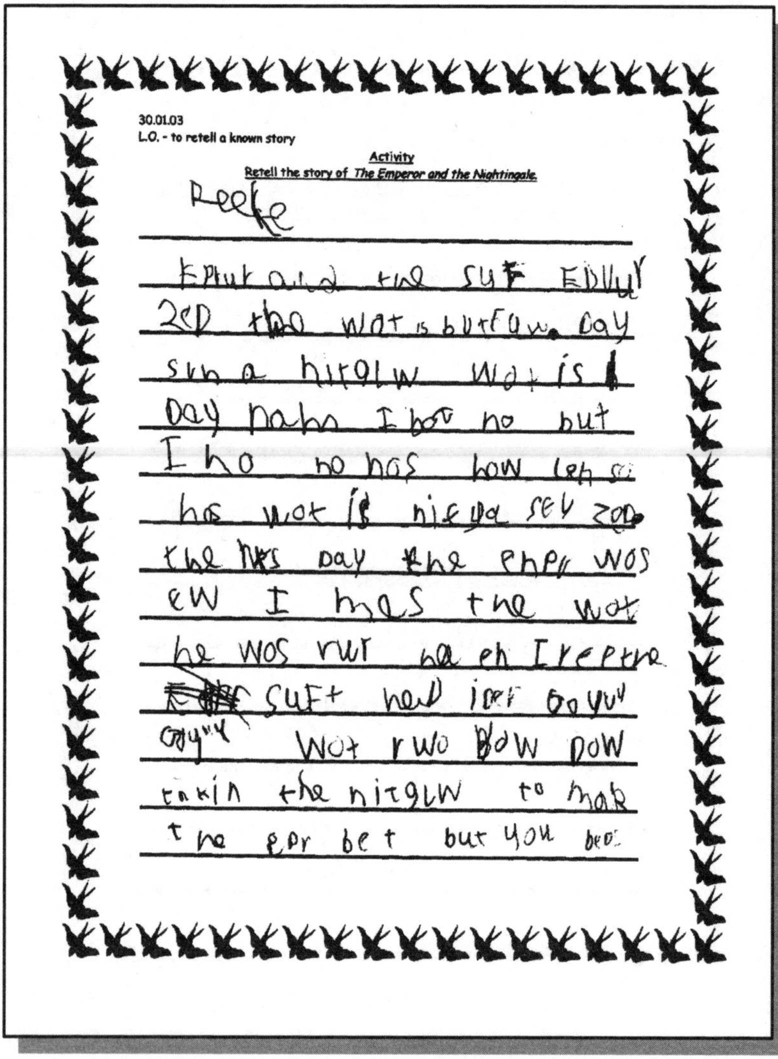
30.01.03

L.O. - to retell a known story

Activity

Retell the story of *The Emperor and the Nightingale.*

Reece

Reece's handwriting after one week of optimum nutrition

Dyslexia Check

Is your child...

☐ ... a relatively late speaker compared to other children of their age?

☐ ... good at things that have a strong visual element, but inexplicably poor in other set tasks?

☐ ... showing evidence of laterality confusion? (Check this by: Asking which hand s/he writes with, which foot s/he takes penalties with, which eye they look through a cardboard tube with. Hand them your watch – which eye do they hold it up to? Does everything happen with the same side or are some things done left-sided and others right-sided?)

☐ ... all right with following a number of instructions in a sequence? For instance, 'Go to the living room and get my slippers, then bring them to me.'

☐ ... writing reversed letters or numbers?

☐ ... having particular difficulty with literacy or one area of literacy, such as spelling or reading?

☐ ... noticeably inconsistent when reading – recognising words, then being unable to read the same word later in the day/book/page?

☐ ... spotting words spelt correctly when offered a range of spellings for the same word?

☐ ... often spelling the same word in different ways on the same page? And if asked the difference between the various spellings, can they identify them?

☐ ... when engaged in literacy tasks, taking a noticeably different time to do them than other tasks, such as drawing or practical activities?

☐ ... able to give an answer verbally or read out a story, but producing little when asked to write it?

☐ ... described by others as clumsy?

☐ ... comfortable with adding a rhyming or alliterative word to a sequence of rhyming or alliterative words?

☐ ... on a much easier reading book than most of their close friends?

☐ ... in a much lower spelling group than their close friends?

☐ ... showing a marked difference compared to the rest of their class during note-taking or a copying activity?

☐ ... showing a noticeable difference in work output if given help with planning their work?

☐ ... producing more work, and generally seeming much happier at school, if taught strategies to develop sequencing skills?

☐ ... beginning to resist writing because they are bad at it?

☐ ... looking up at the board during a copying activity much more often that the children around them (suggesting a weak short-term visual memory)?

☐ ... responding to a handwriting development programme?

☐ ... losing confidence over time in an educational setting?

☐ ... complaining that 'the words move around on the page' when he or she is trying to read?

Tick the box for 'yes'. If you tick a lot of 'yes' boxes, it's best to see an educational psychologist, who can check out if your child has dyslexia.

The eyes have it – omega-3s and vitamin A

Because visual acuity and the ability of the brain to process information from the eye are central to reading and writing, ensuring eye and brain are optimally nourished is important if your child is struggling with these skills. And when it comes to that, oily fish and carrots are the dynamic duo.

While we've now seen how the brain is rich in the omega-3 fats some oily fish are positively swimming in, there is also a concentration of these essential fats in the eyes, along with vitamin A. In fact, so vital is vitamin A to vision that its name, retinol, is a direct reference to its role in keeping the retina working properly. (Retinol is the animal form of vitamin A, found in meat, fish and eggs; beta-carotene, the vegetable form, is converted into retinol in the body.)

Some fish oil supplements – notably cod liver oil – contain

both both vitamin A as retinol and omega-3 fats, so if you suspect your child's problems with reading or writing are down to vision problems, you could try giving them this kind of supplement for a month.

The ideal amount of omega-3, and most specifically DHA and EPA, are given on page 48. With vitamin A, it is vital to know safe limits, as it is one of the few vitamins that can be stored in the body and in very large amounts may cause problems.

During pregnancy, for instance, a woman taking more than 5,000mcg a day may increase the risk of birth defects in her child. For your child, the ideal amount is much less than this – between 500mcg and 2,000mcg, depending on your child's age (see page 250). The table below shows much your child would need to eat to achieve 500mcg.

Vitamin A in Foods

Type of food	Amount giving 500mcg of vitamin A (as retinol)
Liver	4g
Whole milk	160g
Cheddar cheese	160g
Parmesan cheese	240g
Cream cheese	110g
Egg	6 eggs
Butter	11 tablespoons
Mackerel	900g
Kidney	130g
Chicken	1.6kg

Of course, no one is going to eat that much chicken, mackerel, butter or egg at one sitting; but it's important to know how much vitamin A your child's food contains so you can balance that out with all other sources of vitamin A. Most multivitamins will contain some retinol, usually in the region of 500mcg. Cod liver oil capsules vary considerably, however, so do check the label – most will provide between 500 and 1,000mcg per capsule.

You'll need to ensure that the combination of food, supplements and fish oil capsules, added up, doesn't exceed double the optimum daily supplemental amount of vitamin A according to your child's age, shown on page 250. However, do make sure your child is getting both omega-3s and vitamin A.

Pesticides – bad news for the eyes

When the eye is processing visual information, it turns vitamin A into rhodopsin, a light-sensitive pigment. Light reaching the rhodopsin reacts with it, after which the pigment undergoes a cycle of changes that, effectively, recycles it so it turns back into rhodopsin. This cycle is particularly important for black and white vision, which is for the most part what we use at night – hence your grandmother always telling you carrots help you see in the dark.

Organophosphate pesticides and herbicides, now being phased out in most developed countries but still used widely in developing countries, block this conversion. While this is unlikely to be a significant factor in your child's visual ability, it does highlight why it is so important to keep our children free from such chemicals – so keep choosing organic food whenever you can (see Chapter 8).

There are several simple steps you can take to support your child's reading and writing.

- **Ensure an optimum intake of vitamin A from food, supplements and fish oil capsules.**

- **Optimise your child's intake of essential fats, especially omega-3, by giving them flaxseeds, oily fish and/or fish oil supplements every day.**

- **Keep your child 'chemical free' by choosing organic food whenever possible.**

CHAPTER 14

Enhancing Mood and Behaviour

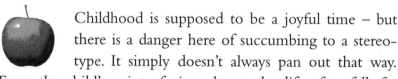 Childhood is supposed to be a joyful time – but there is a danger here of succumbing to a stereotype. It simply doesn't always pan out that way. From the child's point of view, day-to-day life often falls far short of the ideal. Many are no strangers to sadness, boredom, ennui, irritability and anger.

According to research at the University of London and Warwick University, the incidence of depression among young people has doubled over the past 12 years. And over the last 10 years, the number of children on antidepressants has grown steadily to around 40,000, until the virtual ban on giving them to children in 2004, in recognition of their ineffectiveness and the increased risk of suicide associated with them, among other side-effects.

Much better solutions than this are to hand. So if your child is frequently sad or cries a lot, doesn't enjoy or participate in activities, is always bored and has low self-esteem, or is irritable, angry, hostile to others or self-destructive, you can help them. There are two avenues to explore – psychological and biochemical. But as we'll see, they're intimately intertwined.

Getting to the root of unhappiness

Conventionally, anger is not an emotion we are allowed to express, much less our kids. Some children – angry at something happening at school, with their friends or at home – bottle it up as depression. Although you, as a parent, can help tremendously, every child also benefits from having an open, sympathetic adult other than their parents to talk to, to guide them and help them find solutions to their problems. The UK charity Childline, for instance, receives around 2,000 calls each year from children at the brink of their endurance.

One of the greatest unrecognised truths is the role of nutrition in the psychological health of our children. Ensuring your child is optimally nourished will not only improve their mood, but also give them the energy and motivation to deal with life's inevitable ups and downs. Few child psychotherapists and paediatricians recognise how much better their results would be if they helped children tune up their brain biochemistry.

There are a number of common imbalances connected to nutrition that can worsen a child's mood and motivation, some of which will already be familiar:

- Blood sugar imbalances (often associated with excessive sugar and caffeine intake)

- Deficiencies of nutrients (vitamin B3, B6, folate, B12, C, zinc, magnesium, essential fats)

- Deficiencies of tryptophan and tyrosine (precursors of neurotransmitters)

- Allergies and sensitivities.

Poor control of blood glucose levels is a huge factor in low mood, yet a relatively simple aspect of your child's daily routine to fix. As we saw in Chapter 2, you can help them here by always providing breakfast, as well as regular meals and snacks composed of natural, unprocessed foods. But what about those key nutrients?

Beating the blues with nutrition

Among nutrients, the most promising for improving mood are vitamins B3, B12 and folic acid, then vitamin B6, zinc and magnesium and the essential fats (especially omega-3s, which we discussed in detail in Chapter 3). Most of these are involved in the biochemical process known as methylation, which is critical for balancing the neurotransmitters that keep your child motivated and happy. Improved methylation is also associated with better grades at school.

The B connection

Folic acid is found in green leafy vegetables, nuts, seeds and beans. Far too many children have far too few of these, yet their effect can be astounding – as an intriguing study by Bernard Gesch has shown.

Gesch wondered what the effect of giving B vitamins and essential fats to Britain's worst young offenders would be. After persuading the UK Home Office to allow the first UK double-blind trial on young offenders in a maximum security prison in Aylesbury, he gave them either a multinutrient containing vitamins, minerals and essential fats, or a placebo. The results, published in the *British Journal of Psychiatry*, showed a staggering 35 per cent decrease in acts of aggression in the prisoners eating the multi after only two weeks.[106]

Since prison diets are, if anything, already better than those most of these young people ate at home, this shows just how important optimum nutrition is for reducing violent and deviant behaviour. When the trial was over and the supplements were stopped, there was a 40 per cent increase in offences in the prison.

Magnesium – relaxing mind and muscle

Gesch also gave magnesium and zinc to the young offenders in his study. These two minerals are among the most important for mental health – we've seen how zinc, for instance, helps with problems such as confusion, depression and slow mental processing. Magnesium has a relaxant effect on both mind and muscles, and deficiencies are very common, manifesting as muscle aches, cramps and spasms, as well as anxiety, irritability, hyperactivity and insomnia. Children often have low levels, which can be helped via supplementation.

A child needs between 250 and 500mg of magnesium a day. Seeds and nuts are rich in magnesium, as are vegetables and fruit, especially dark green leafy vegetables such as kale or spinach. We recommend that children eat these magnesium-rich foods every day and supplement an additional 50 to 100mg of magnesium.

Fats to fight depression

We've already encountered omega-3 fish oils in a number of contexts. And as it happens, they are very much part of the equation for happiness. The better a child's blood levels of omega-3 fats, the better their levels of serotonin – the 'happy' neurotransmitter – are likely to be. The reason for this is that omega-3 fats help build the brain's receptor sites for serotonin, as well as improving reception. According to Dr Joseph Hibbeln, who discovered that fish eaters are less prone to depression, 'It's like building more serotonin factories, instead of just increasing the efficiency of the serotonin you have.'[107]

Many trials have now been published proving that omega-3 fats are highly effective as a treatment for depression.[108] EPA is the top omega-3 for this job.

A case in point is a small-scale study by Dr Basant Puri from London's Hammersmith Hospital. Puri decided to try ethyl-EPA on one of his patients, a 21-year-old student who had been on a variety of antidepressants, to no avail. He had a very low sense of self-esteem, sleeping problems, little appetite, found it hard to socialise and often thought of killing himself. After a month of supplementing omega-3 fats, he was no longer having suicidal thoughts and after nine months no longer had any depression.[109] Trials on younger children are currently underway and are also likely to prove effective.

Balancing act – neurotransmitters and mood

There are often two sides to feeling low – feeling miserable, and feeling apathetic and unmotivated. The most prevalent theory for the cause of these imbalances is a brain imbalance in two families of neurotransmitters, the molecules of emotion. These are:

- Serotonin, which influences your mood

- Adrenalin and noradrenalin, made from dopamine, which influence your motivation.

But this imbalance isn't just about nutrition. Let's look at some of the other factors in your child's life that could be fuelling any unhappiness and apathy they're experiencing.

Stresses and strains – how imbalance sets in

The mad, goal-driven dash of 21st-century living can be very stressful for children. Too many children are pressured to perform in a century where the motto is 'succeed and achieve'. Perhaps living out their parent's dissatisfactions, they go from school to piano lessons to extra coaching, with no time left to simply do nothing, dream or play.

All this has an inevitable effect on the brain, which produces more and more adrenalin and serotonin in response to the too frequent ups and downs, and numerous stresses and strains. It's akin to the body's production of more and more insulin to even out frequently fluctuating blood sugar levels. This increases a child's need for the building blocks, the amino acids, from which we make these mood-enhancing neurotransmitters. Combine these psychological pressures with the all-too-common poor diet, and too many children go over the edge into low moods and erratic behaviour.

Over the last few years, what has been learnt about both serotonin, the 'happy' neurotransmitter, and adrenalin and noradrenalin, 'the motivators', is that there are four main reasons for deficiency in children, in addition to a lack of amino acids. These are:

• Not enough light

• Not enough exercise

• Too much stress

• Not enough co-factor B vitamins, zinc and magnesium.

So – if your child is melancholy or depressed, misbehaving, exhausted, tends to comfort eat and is experiencing disturbed sleep patterns, the chances are that a combination of factors are working together to leave them short on serotonin, noradrenalin or adrenalin.

How does it happen? Light is very important as a brain stimulator, yet with our increasingly indoor lives most of us don't get enough of it. The difference in light exposure outside and inside is massive. Many of us spend 23 out of 24 hours a day indoors, exposed to an average of 100 units (called lux) of light. Compare that to the 20,000 lux of a sunny day, and 7,000 lux of an overcast day. So most of us are simply not exposing ourselves to enough direct sunlight to maximise serotonin production. And of course, it's worse in winter when the days are shorter.

Stress – say, from exams or bullying – also rapidly reduces serotonin levels and also raises adrenalin, leading to burnout. A couch-potato habit can make this worse because physical exercise improves the stress response, and reduces the stress-induced depletion of serotonin and adrenalin. Exercise itself is an incredibly powerful mood booster.

The message is that you need to ensure your child has the time and opportunity to play outdoors for a reasonable time each day, and get daily exercise.

Supplementing for neurotransmitter balance

You might find that your child needs extra help in recovering from difficulties with mood. In these cases, look to supplementation: there are a number of possibilities.

Go for the right amino acids

Serotonin is made from a constituent of protein, the amino acid tryptophan. Dr Philip Cowen from Oxford University's psychiatry department has proven that if you deprive adults of tryptophan, most experience a worsening of mood and start to show signs of depression within seven hours.[110] Tryptophan is especially abundant in fish, turkey, chicken, cheese, beans, tofu, oats and eggs. A child's diet, depending on age, needs to contain between 500mg and 1,000mg of tryptophan a day, which they can easily achieve by eating one or two of the following meals, each giving 500mg of it:

- Oat porridge, soya milk and two scrambled eggs

- Baked potato with cottage cheese and tuna salad

- Chicken breast, potatoes au gratin and green beans

- Wholewheat spaghetti with bean, tofu or meat sauce

- Salmon fillet, quinoa and lentil pilaf, and green salad with yoghurt dressing.

Adrenalin and noradrenalin are made from the food amino acids called phenylalanine and tyrosine. These are also found in protein foods – the same kind that are rich in tryptophan. So ensuring adequate protein intake, as we saw in Chapter 5, helps keep your child's mood and motivation positive.

In adult studies, supplementing 5-hydroxy-tryptophan (5-HTP), the amino acid from which the body makes serotonin, along with tyrosine, the amino acid from which the body

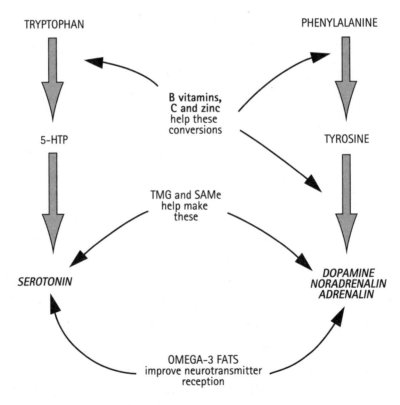

How nutrients affect mood boosting neurotransmitters

makes adrenalin and noradrenalin, has proven highly effective in correcting mood problems.

There have been 27 studies to date, giving adults between 100 and 900mg a day, showing 5-HTP to be highly effective in restoring a balanced mood, without any significant side-effects. The worst that seems to happen is that, in very large doses, some people become nauseated. For children, depending on age, supplement between 20 and 50mg of 5-HTP. Not only is 5-HTP a highly effective mood booster, much more so than antidepressants, it also has no significant side-effects.[111]

Try TMG – the master tuner

In the figure on page 142 you might have noticed two strange-sounding nutrients: TMG or tri-methyl glycine, and SAMe (s-adenosyl methionine). Both are amino acids that help to keep the brain and nervous system well tuned by donating so-called methyl groups. These are important in the transformation of neurotransmitters. For example, noradrenalin turns into adrenalin by having a methyl group added. This process of adding on methyl groups, and sometimes taking them away, is crucial to the task of keeping the brain in balance.

SAMe is one of the most comprehensively studied natural antidepressants. Over 100 placebo-controlled, double-blind studies show that SAMe is equal to or superior to antidepressants, and works faster – most often within a few days (most pharmaceutical antidepressants may take three to six weeks to take effect), and with few side-effects.[112–114]

While SAMe is classified as a medicine, TMG, the amino acid from which it is made, is a component of food, and is especially high in roots and sprouts. So eating carrots, parsnips, beetroot, turnip, swedes, potato and beansprouts will provide your child with TMG. Although it's not classified as an essential nutrient, we recommend that children eat at least

100mg a day, which translates as a serving of a root vegetable or sprout.

To help children with behavioural problems and low mood, give them supplements with all of these amino acids – 5-HTP, phenylalanine or tyrosine, TMG – together with the B vitamins that help turn them into neurotransmitters (B3, B6, B12 and folic acid). Some children's formulas contain these nutrients, which literally help the brain connect properly (see Resources for details).

At the Brain Bio Centre, we test children for their blood levels of essential fats, serotonin, adrenalin and noradrenalin, as well as homocysteine, which tells whether a child needs more B vitamins and TMG. From that we can devise the perfect nutrition programme of food and supplements to help them achieve their full potential.

Fourteen-year-old Liam had been kicked out of mainstream school for disruptive behaviour. His homocysteine score was 24 – the average for a 90-year-old! One month of B vitamins, magnesium, TMG and omega-3 supplements later, along with a low-sugar diet, brought his level down to 9. In his own words:

'After about 10 days after starting the diet and the vitamins I noticed I was less tired in the morning. Now I'm not tired at all when I wake up. I have loads more energy, I'm less bored, I'm concentrating better and I feel a lot happier. I'm getting on better at school and concentrating better in class. I'm also doing more activities and sports. I feel better, having got my homocysteine level down. I feel more positive about my future. Since starting the diet I'm a lot calmer than I used to be and I haven't got into trouble at all. I'm going to stay on the diet for life and keep taking the vitamins. It's brilliant!'

To keep your child's mood, motivation and behaviour good, do the following.

- Give them a diet containing protein-rich foods (fish, meat, eggs, pulses) and TMG-rich foods (root vegetables and sprouts).

- Optimise your child's intake of essential fats, especially omega-3 fats, by giving them flaxseeds, oily fish and/or fish oil supplements every day.

- Ensure optimum nutrition with a good multivitamin providing all the B vitamins, plus magnesium and zinc.

- If your child is low in energy, mood or motivation or is under stress, underperforming or acting up, give them an additional supplement containing TMG, 5-HTP, tyrosine or phenylalanine.

PART 3

Solving Problems

Are children today having a 'kid-life crisis'? Mental health problems are very much on the increase in children – from autism and learning difficulties to hyperactivity and aggression. A major reason for these increases is often sub-optimum nutrition. In this part we give you nutritional solutions to these and other problems to help you maximise your child's potential for mental and emotional health and happiness.

CHAPTER 15

Dyslexia and Dyspraxia – What Works

 Nowadays, any child with learning and behavioural problems tends to get put into one of a number of boxes. Are they dyslexic, having problems with words and writing? Are they dyspraxic, having problems with coordination? Do they have 'attention deficit hyperactivity disorder' (ADHD), the official term for what used to be known as hyperactivity but still denotes poor attention span, concentration and hyperactive behaviour?

In most children who have problems with learning or behaviour, there are substantial overlaps between these categories. While a minority of children are purely dyslexic, more will show features of two, three or all of these conditions in differing degrees of severity. Around half the dyslexic population is likely to be dyspraxic, and vice versa, and the mutual overlap between ADHD and dyslexia/dyspraxia is also around 50 per cent.[115] But unfortunately, it's rare to find diagnosis or treatment that take account of these complexities. ADHD, for instance, lies firmly in the realm of psychiatry, and is usually treated with stimulant medication (see Chapter 16).

Current evidence suggests that up to 20 per cent of the population may be affected to some degree by one or more of

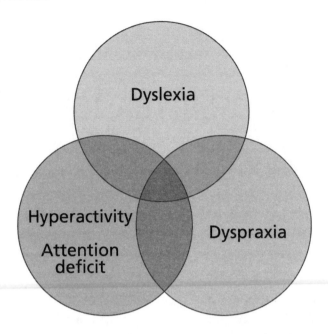

Dyslexia, dyspraxia and attention deficit hyperactive disorder overlap

these conditions. The associated difficulties usually persist into adulthood, causing serious problems not only for those affected but for society as a whole.

Is your child affected?

Children with dyslexia experience specific problems in learning to read and write, sometimes because of subtle variations in visual perception. Difficulties in arithmetic and reading musical notation are also common, as are poor working memory, problems with deciphering the sounds of words, and a faulty sense of direction.

Around 5 per cent of the population is severely dyslexic, although many more are affected by milder forms of the condition. If you suspect your child might be dyslexic, begin by completing the Dyslexia Check in Chapter 13, page 131. Many schools have special-needs teachers who can assess your child thoroughly. If your child's school doesn't do this, contact the Dyslexia Institute (see Resources, page 278); they can put you in touch with an educational psychologist who can carry out this assessment.

Getting your child assessed is useful on a number of counts: it helps them become aware that they have a difficulty, allows them to work with a special-needs teacher to minimise the problem, and gives them special privileges such as more time for exams and the use of computers at school.

Recent research suggests that pure dyslexia – that is, substantially delayed reading and writing in otherwise bright children – may have to do with a subtle brain difference in how these children perceive the 'small sounds', or phonetical building blocks, of words. This makes it harder for them to both read and understand word meanings, as they simply don't have a good grip on the basics. Special teaching techniques to compensate for this can dramatically improve your child's reading and writing skills. The Dyslexia Institute can help you locate a teacher.

Less well known but equally prevalent, dyspraxia involves poor coordination and difficulties in carrying out complex sequenced actions. Children with the condition find it hard catching a ball, tying up shoelaces or doing up buttons, but more seriously, their handwriting can be extremely difficult to read, and they can experience real difficulties with organisation, attention and concentration.

Eat for vision and coordination

On top of assessments and tailored teaching, children with dyslexia and dyspraxia can benefit massively from the right nutrition. Again, it's all down to nutrients that will help brain and eyes.

Essential fats – seeing is believing

We discussed the importance of essential fats for proper brain function in Chapter 4. Children with dyslexia, dyspraxia and learning difficulties are very often deficient in these essential fats and/or the nutrients needed to properly utilise them, and the benefits of increasing the intake of these fats have been clearly documented in many studies.[116–117] A high concentration of essential fats is needed in the eyes before they can manage the very rapid movements associated with vision.

A study of 97 dyslexic children by Dr Alex Richardson and colleagues at Hammersmith Hospital in London revealed that essential fat deficiency clearly contributes to the severity of dyslexic problems. Those children with the worst essential fat deficiencies showed significantly poorer reading and lower general ability than the non-deficient children.[118]

How do you know if your child is deficient in essential fats? You could start with the Fat Check in Chapter 3 (see page 40). A key indicator is dry skin or eczema, and in a study of 60 children at the Royal London Hospital, Dr Christine Absolon and colleagues found twice the rate of 'psychological disturbance' in children with eczema, compared to those without.[119]

If your child has some of the outward symptoms of essential fat deficiency – rough dry patches on the skin, cracked lips, dull or dry hair, soft or brittle nails, and excessive thirst – it is fair to say that this could be an underlying factor in learning difficulties they might be experiencing, such as concentration or visual problems, mood swings, disturbed sleep patterns and in some cases behavioural problems. This is because dyslexia, dyspraxia, learning difficulties and ADHD all involve poor nerve cell communications in the brain, and essential fats are crucial in keeping neurons talking to each other.[120]

To test the value of supplementing essential fats in dyspraxia, Dr Jacqueline Stordy of the University of Surrey in the UK gave essential fat supplements containing DHA, EPA, AA and

DGLA to 15 children whose performance on standardised measures of motor and coordination skills placed them in the bottom 1 per cent of the population. After 12 weeks of supplementation, they all showed significant improvements in manual dexterity, ball skills, balance and parental ratings of their dyspraxic symptoms.[121]

Stordy also assessed the benefit of essential fat supplementation in dyslexia, and found that after just four weeks of supplementation with EPA and DHA, their night vision and dark adaptation (which are usually very poor in dyslexics) had completely normalised.[122]

Of course, it's just as vital for kids with dyslexia and dyspraxia to avoid fried and hydrogenated fats as to top up their essential fats.

The copper–zinc link

While much of the current research into nutritional solutions for dyslexia and dyspraxia is focusing on essential fats, some scientists are looking at copper – a potentially toxic element reported to be high in dyslexic children.[123] Since zinc and vitamin C are both antagonists of copper, this is another possible explanation for their reported benefits.

Along with the recommendations in Chapter 13, we suggest you take the following steps if your child is dyslexic or dyspraxic.

- **Ensure they're getting an optimal intake of nutrients from their diet as well as a good-quality multivitamin/mineral supplement with enough zinc.**

- **Minimise your child's intake of sugar and refined or processed foods that provide ample calories but few nutrients, and encourage them to eat more nutrient-rich foods.**

- Ensure an optimal intake of essential fats from seeds, their cold-pressed oils and oily fish, plus sufficient anti-oxidants, especially vitamin E, to protect them from free-radical damage.

- Minimise your child's intake of fried food, processed food and saturated fat from meat and dairy.

CHAPTER 16

Drug-Free Solutions for ADHD

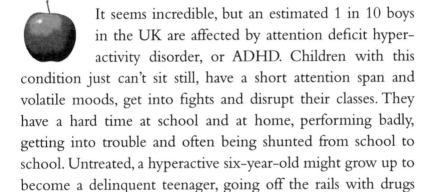 It seems incredible, but an estimated 1 in 10 boys in the UK are affected by attention deficit hyperactivity disorder, or ADHD. Children with this condition just can't sit still, have a short attention span and volatile moods, get into fights and disrupt their classes. They have a hard time at school and at home, performing badly, getting into trouble and often being shunted from school to school. Untreated, a hyperactive six-year-old might grow up to become a delinquent teenager, going off the rails with drugs and alcohol.

At a cursory glance, ADHD might look like something to be blamed on poor parenting or schooling. But dig deeper, and a plethora of other potential causative factors emerges: heredity, smoking, alcohol or drug use during their mothers' pregnancy, oxygen deprivation at birth, prenatal trauma and environmental pollution.

The good news is that more often than not, children with ADHD have one or more nutritional imbalances. Identifying and correcting these can dramatically improve the children's energy, focus, concentration and behaviour.

Eight-year-old Robert is a case in point. Diagnosed with ADHD, he was 'out of control' and his parents were at their wits' end. Robert had also been constipated his entire life. Through biochemical testing at the Brain Bio Centre we found that he was allergic to dairy products and eggs and was very deficient in magnesium. Dietary analysis revealed that he took in excessive amounts of sugar every day. We recommended cutting down his sugar intake significantly, cutting out dairy and egg products and supplementing magnesium and omega-3 essential fats. Within three months, his parents reported that Robert was a different child. He had calmed down considerably and had become much more manageable both at home and at school. His constipation had also cleared completely.

It can be difficult to draw the line between the behaviour of a child that is within the normal limits of high energy, and abnormally active behaviour. Use the checklist below to assess your child, scoring 2 if a symptom is severe, 1 if moderate and 0 if not present. A score below 12 is normal. If it's higher, read on to discover workable nutritional strategies.

Hyperactivity Check

Is your child...

- [ ] ... overactive
- [ ] ... fidgety
- [ ] ... unable to sit still at meals
- [ ] ... too talkative
- [ ] ... clumsy
- [ ] ... unpredictable
- [ ] ... unable to respond to discipline
- [ ] ... displaying speech problems
- [ ] ... unable to listen to a story to the end
- [ ] ... prone to leave projects unfinished
- [ ] ... wearing out toys, furniture, etc.
- [ ] ... uninterested in staying with games
- [ ] ... failing to follow directions
- [ ] ... fighting with other children
- [ ] ... teasing
- [ ] ... 'getting into things'
- [ ] ... having temper tantrums

☐ ... hard to get to bed   ☐ ... defiant
☐ ... reckless   ☐ ... irritable
☐ ... impatient   ☐ ... unpopular with peers
☐ ... accident-prone   ☐ ... lying
☐ ... destructive   ☐ ... wetting the bed

Eat to calm down

If your child has ADHD and is eating poorly, the way is clear: you'll need to take a very close look at the amount of refined carbohydrates, harmful trans fats and other problem foods they're consuming, look at what's missing, and provide a menu designed to calm them down.

Show sugar the door

In Chapter 2 we saw how vital balanced blood sugar levels are to mental health, and advocated a low- or no-sugar diet. A diet high in refined carbohydrates is not good for anyone, but in some children sweet-eating seems to promote hyperactivity and aggression.

Essentially, if you feed your child rocket fuel (that is, sugar and caffeine), don't be surprised if their behaviour is out of control. Even so-called 'normal' children can become uncontrollable after a sugarfest. Dietary studies consistently reveal that hyperactive children eat more sugar than other children,[124] and reducing sugar has been found to halve disciplinary actions in young offenders.[125]

Other research has confirmed that the problem is not sugar itself but the forms it comes in, the absence of a well-balanced diet overall, and abnormal glucose metabolism. A study of 265 hyperactive children found that more than three-quarters of them displayed abnormal glucose tolerance[126] – that is, their bodies were less able to handle sugar intake and maintain balanced blood sugar levels.

In any case, when a child is regularly snacking on refined carbohydrates, sweets, chocolate, fizzy drinks, juices and little or no fibre to slow the glucose absorption, the levels of glucose in their blood will seesaw continually and trigger wild fluctuations in their levels of activity, concentration, focus and behaviour. These, of course, are also the symptoms of ADHD. The initial calm that sometimes sets in after children eat refined carbohydrates may well be a short-lived normalisation of blood sugar levels from a hypoglycemic (low blood sugar) state, during which the brain – including those parts of it that control behaviour – were starved of fuel.

Since children with hyperactivity and ADHD seem particularly sensitive to sugar, it's recommended that you remove all forms of refined sugar and any foods that contain it from their diet. This includes processed juices and juice drinks – these deliver a big shot of sugar very quickly. Replace these with wholefoods and complex carbohydrates such as brown rice and other whole grains, oats, lentils, beans, quinoa and vegetables, which should be eaten throughout the day; three substantial meals and several snacks will keep blood sugar trickling in slowly and evenly.

To further slow the progress of glucose to their bloodstream, you should ensure that your child's intake of carbohydrates is balanced with protein, so that they eat half as much protein as carbohydrates at every meal and snack. For instance, give them a handful of seeds and nuts with a piece of fruit, or have chicken or fish with rice for dinner.

Pump up the essential fats

As we saw in Chapter 12, essential fats are crucial for concentration. Omega-3s in particular have a clearly calming effect on many children with hyperactivity and ADHD. And many children with ADHD, like those with dyslexia, have visible symptoms of essential fat deficiency such as excessive thirst, dry skin, eczema and asthma.

It is also interesting that boys, whose requirement for essential fats is much higher than girls', are also much more likely to have ADHD: four out of five sufferers are male. Researchers have theorised that ADHD children may be deficient in essential fats not just because their dietary intake from foods such as seeds and nuts is inadequate (though this is not uncommon), but also because their need is higher, their absorption is poor, or they are unable to convert these fats well into EPA and DHA, and from DHA into prostaglandins, which are also important for brain function.[127]

So it's of interest that the conversion of essential fats can be inhibited by most of the foods that cause symptoms in children with ADHD, such as wheat, dairy and foods containing salicylates. (More on salicylates later in this chapter.) This conversion is also hindered by deficiencies of the various vitamins and minerals that help the enzymes driving these conversions – vitamin B3 (niacin), B6, C, biotin, zinc and magnesium. Zinc and magnesium deficiency are common in children with ADHD.

Research carried out at Purdue University in the US confirmed that children with ADHD have an inadequate intake of the nutrients required for the conversion of essential fats into prostaglandins, and have lower levels of EPA, DHA, and AA than children without ADHD.[128] Supplementation with all these omega-3 essential fats, pre-converted, along with the omega-6 essential fat GLA, reduced ADHD symptoms such as anxiety, attention difficulties and general behaviour problems.[129–131]

Research at Oxford University has proven the value of these essential fats in a double-blind trial involving 41 children aged 8 to 12 years who had ADHD symptoms and specific learning difficulties. Those children receiving extra essential fats in supplements were both behaving and learning better within 12 weeks.[132] The case study below, courtesy of the Hyperactive Children's Support Group, is revealing in this context.

Six-year-old Stephen had a history of hyperactivity, with severely disturbed sleep and disruptive behaviour at home and at school. Threatened with expulsion from school because of his impossible behaviour, his parents were given two weeks to improve matters. They contacted the Hyperactive Children's Support Group, and evening primrose oil was suggested. Since Stephen was too young for capsules and wouldn't take the oil off a spoon, a dose of 1.5g was rubbed into his skin morning and evening. The school was unaware of this, but after five days the teacher telephoned the mother to say that never, in 30 years of teaching, had she seen such a dramatic change in a child's behaviour.

After three weeks the evening primrose oil was stopped, and one week later the school again complained. The oil was then reintroduced, and again its effect clearly showed in Stephen's improved behaviour. It's worth noting that rubbing oil on the skin is not nearly as effective as taking it by mouth, because only a small percentage of it makes it into the body – so Stephen's story is all the more remarkable.

Many children do not eat rich sources of omega-3 essential fats, and could benefit from eating more oily fish (wild or organic salmon, sardines, mackerel, fresh tuna) and seeds such as flax, hemp, sunflower and pumpkin or their cold-pressed oils. It is also important to replace foods known to hinder the conversion of essential fats to prostaglandins – such as deep-fried foods – while supplementing the nutrients needed for the conversion, such as B vitamins and zinc, as discussed above.

Sort out the allergies

Of all the avenues so far explored, the link between hyperactivity and food sensitivity is the most established and worthy of pursuit in any child showing signs of ADHD.

A study by Dr Joseph Bellanti of Georgetown University in

Washington DC found that hyperactive children are seven times more likely to have food allergies than other children. According to his research, 56 per cent of hyperactive children aged 7 to 10 tested positive for food allergies, compared to less than 8 per cent of 'normal' children. A separate investigation by the Hyperactive Children's Support Group found that 89 per cent of children with ADHD reacted to food colourings, 72 per cent to flavourings, 60 per cent to MSG, 45 per cent to all synthetic additives, 50 per cent to cow's milk, 60 per cent to chocolate and 40 per cent to oranges.[133] (For more on food additives, see Chapter 8.)

Other substances often found to induce behavioural changes are wheat, corn, yeast, soya, peanuts and eggs.[134] Symptoms strongly linked to allergy include nasal problems and excessive mucus, ear infections, facial swelling and discoloration around the eyes, tonsillitis, digestive problems, bad breath, eczema, asthma, headaches and bedwetting. (See Chapter 9 for more details on identifying and eliminating food allergies in your child.)

Up to 90 per cent of hyperactive children benefit from eliminating foods that contain artificial colours, flavours and preservatives; processed and manufactured foods; and 'culprit' foods identified by either an exclusion diet or blood test.[135] Some parents have also reported success with the Feingold diet, removing not only all artificial additives but also foods that naturally contain compounds called salicylates.

Researchers at the University of Sydney in Australia found that three-quarters of 86 children with ADHD reacted adversely to foods containing salicylates.[136] These include prunes, raisins, raspberries, almonds, apricots, canned cherries, blackcurrants, oranges, strawberries, grapes, tomato sauce, plums, cucumbers and Granny Smith apples. As the list of foods containing salicylates is very long and contains many otherwise nutritious foods, cutting them all out should be considered only as a secondary course of action, and must be carefully planned and monitored by a nutritional therapist.

Understanding how a low-salicylate diet helps hyperactive children does offer a useful alternative to such a drastic course of action. Salicylates inhibit the conversion and utilisation of essential fats, which we know are often low in hyperactive children. So instead of avoiding salicylates, it may help to simply increase the supply of essential fats – and as we've seen, that has indeed been shown to work.

Fix the deficiencies

As we've now seen abundantly, studies have shown that academic performance improves and behavioural problems diminish significantly when children are given nutritional supplements. Although it is unlikely, on the basis of the studies to date, that ADHD is purely a deficiency disease, most children with this diagnosis *are* deficient in certain key nutrients, and do respond very well.

Zinc and magnesium are the most commonly deficient nutrients in people with ADHD. In fact, symptoms of deficiency in these minerals are very similar to the symptoms of ADHD. Low levels of magnesium, for instance, can cause excessive fidgeting, anxious restlessness, insomnia, coordination problems and learning difficulties (if accompanied by a normal IQ).

Polish researchers studying 116 children with ADHD for their levels of magnesium found that 95 per cent of them were deficient in it – a much higher percentage than that among healthy children. The team also noted a correlation between levels of magnesium and severity of symptoms. Supplementing 200mg of magnesium for six months significantly reduced hyperactivity in the children with ADHD, but behaviour in the control group, who received no magnesium, worsened.[137]

Dr Neil Ward of the University of Surrey has come up with

a finding that could explain the link between ADHD and such deficiencies. In a study of 530 hyperactive children, Ward found that compared to children without ADHD, a significantly higher percentage of children with the condition had had several courses of antibiotics in early childhood.[138] Further investigations revealed that children who had had three or more such courses before the age of three tested for significantly lower levels of zinc, calcium, chromium and selenium.[139] This is probably because antibiotics have a disruptive effect on beneficial gut flora and consequently on overall digestive health, as discussed in Chapter 9.

Even without supplements, tailoring a child's diet to include higher levels of key nutrients can lead to significant improvements in behaviour. Dr Stephen Schoenthaler of the Department of Social and Criminal Justice at California State University, Stanislaus, has conducted extensive investigations into the relationship between poor diet, nutrient status and bad behaviour.

In his many placebo-controlled studies conducted over 18 months in Alabama, Florida and Virginia, which involved over 1,000 long-term young offenders, Schoenthaler discovered that introducing a better diet improved behaviour by between 40 and 60 per cent. Blood tests for vitamins and minerals showed that around a third of the young people involved had low levels of one or more vitamins and minerals before the trial, but that by the end of the study, some 70 to 90 per cent of those whose levels had risen demonstrated a massive improvement in behaviour.[140]

Kick out the toxic nasties

Looking beyond low levels of essential nutrients, excess anti-nutrients can also induce ADHD symptoms. An example of this is copper, which is found in high levels in some children with ADHD. Studies have also revealed a link between high aluminium and hyperactivity. Many toxic elements deplete the body of essential nutrients such as zinc, and may contribute to nutritional deficiencies. A hair mineral analysis to rule out heavy metal intoxication is therefore an important component of an overall nutritional approach. See Chapter 7 for more on how to get heavy metals out of your child's system.

The rise of Ritalin

It's a sad fact that many hyperactive children are never evaluated for chemical, nutritional or allergic factors, nor are they treated nutritionally. Instead, when faced with a child who has ADHD, most doctors typically write out a prescription for a habit-forming amphetamine such as Ritalin or Concerta, which have many properties similar to those of cocaine. In fact, using brain imaging techniques, Dr Nora Volkow of the Brookhaven National Laboratory in Upton, New York, has shown that Ritalin is actually more potent than cocaine. So why has prescribing it so widely not produced an army of addicted schoolchildren? Volkow has revealed that it's because it takes about an hour for Ritalin in pill form to affect the brain, while smoked or injected cocaine works in seconds.[141]

Despite these findings, the flood of Ritalin prescriptions shows no sign of abating. Ritalin is now given to up to 20 per cent of children in some American schools, even though researchers looking at its effectiveness have found that it can worsen the behaviour of more children than it helps.

In 2004, prescriptions for Ritalin and other methylphenidate drugs had risen to 360,000, at a cost of £12.5 million. That's double the level prescribed in 1999. And this is only one type of stimulant drug prescribed to children.[142] In the US, more than 8 million children are now on the drug – that's a staggering 10 per cent of all boys between the ages of 6 and 14. Other drugs that are used are slight variations on Ritalin – for example, sustained-release versions. A newer drug, Strattera (atomoxetine), is also prescribed for ADHD. It works by preventing the reuptake of the neurotransmitter noradrenalin, thus keeping more of it in circulation.

It's thought that the calming effect of drugs like Ritalin and Strattera on hyperactive children is because there is not enough of the neurotransmitter noradrenalin in the part of the brain that is supposed to filter out unimportant stimuli. Dr Joan Baizer at the University of Buffalo in upstate New York has shown that while Ritalin was previously thought to have only short-term effects, it actually initiates changes in brain structure and function that remain long after the therapeutic effects have dissipated.[143]

Dr Peter Breggin, a psychiatrist at the International Center for the Study of Psychiatry and Psychology in the US, is an outspoken critic of Ritalin. He says the drug, far from helping children with ADHD, actually damages the brain of the developing child by decreasing blood flow. 'Ritalin does not correct biochemical imbalances – it causes them,' he says, further alleging that negative research results are being suppressed to protect the enormous profits from the drug's sale.

This is not good news when you consider the US Drug Enforcement Agency's list of side-effects from this drug. On top of increased blood pressure, heart rate, respiration and temperature, people taking Ritalin can experience appetite suppression, stomach pains, weight loss, growth retardation, facial tics, muscle twitching, euphoria, nervousness, irritability, agitation, insomnia, psychotic episodes, violent behaviour, paranoid delusions, hallucinations, bizarre behaviours, heart arrhythmias and palpitations, psychological dependence and even death.[144]

Nor does Ritalin work over time. The US National Institutes of Health concluded that there is no evidence of any long-term improvement in scholastic performance on Ritalin.[145]

What's more, a child given Ritalin or other stimulant drugs is more likely to become addicted to smoking and abuse other stimulant substances later in life, such as cocaine. The long and short of it is – don't accept a prescription for these drugs on behalf of your child.[146]

Given the possible effect of Ritalin on noradrenalin deficiency in the brain, it is interesting to note that magnesium plays a key role in promoting the production of noradrenalin. And sure enough, the vast majority of children are able to stop taking Ritalin after as little as three weeks once they start supplementing 500mg of magnesium daily. While giving your child up to 200mg of magnesium is perfectly safe, we don't recommend larger amounts unless you are under the guidance of a nutritional therapist. Other nutrients also involved in the production of noradrenalin include manganese, iron, copper, zinc, vitamin C and vitamin B6,[147] and many of these nutrients are also involved in the proper metabolism of essential fats (see below).

Despite the tremendous results reported for nutritional approaches to ADHD, Ritalin is far more commonly prescribed than supplements. Dr Bernard Rimland assessed the relative efficacy of different nutrient strategies compared to drugs such as Ritalin, and found that supplementing B6 and magnesium was 10 times more effective than Ritalin!

Vitamins vs drugs – which work best for ADHD?

After Dr Bernard Rimland looked at how well a nutritional approach to ADHD works in a study with 191 children, the late Humphry Osmond, a doctor based in Saskatchewan, Canada, decided to compare this to results with drugs. Osmond reported the total number of children taking each drug, the number helped, the number worsened and the 'relative efficacy ratio' – that is, the

---

number helped divided by the number worsened. So if twice as many are helped as worsened, the ratio is 2. If the same numbers of people are helped as worsened, the ratio is 1.

The results showed that as many ADHD sufferers are worsened by medication as are helped. In stark contrast, 18 times as many sufferers are helped rather than harmed with a nutritional approach, with 66 per cent responding positively.

ADHD Treatments – Comparing the Results

Medication	Total	No. Helped	No. Worsened	Relative Efficacy Ratio
Dexedrine	172	44	80	0.55
Ritalin	66	22	27	0.81
Mysoline	10	4	4	1.00
Valium	106	31	31	1.00
Dilantin	204	57	43	1.33
Benadril	151	34	25	1.36
Stelazine	120	40	28	1.43
Deanol	73	17	10	1.70
Mellaril	277	101	55	1.84
All drugs	1,591	440	425	1.04
Vitamins	191	127	7	18.14

As you can see from the box above, the best drug against ADHD was Mellaril, not Ritalin. However, neither of these drugs were as effective as vitamin B6 and magnesium or the brain nutrient DMAE, prescribed as Deanol in the US, which was also twice as effective as Ritalin (see page 168).

While there is much you can do yourself, ADHD is a complex condition. As such, it really demands supervision and treatment by a qualified practitioner, who can devise the correct nutritional strategy for your child. Your child's supplement requirements must be individually assessed, and they will need to follow an optimally healthy diet. A minimum of three to six months will probably pass before you see any substantial results, but you may well see a general slowing down from hyperactivity and improved concentration in your child very quickly. As your child starts to feel and behave better, the positive feedback they receive from their parents and teachers can encourage them to stick to the nutritional programme long term – which is what really produces the best results.

Reward deficiency syndrome

Some children with ADHD also suffer from 'reward deficiency syndrome',[148] where they have a constant need for stimulation. This is thought to happen because they either don't produce enough of the motivating neurotransmitter dopamine (from which adrenalin and noradrenalin are made), or don't respond strongly enough to their own dopamine.

Drugs like cocaine and Ritalin both increase dopamine production and dopamine sensitivity, at least in the short term. For these children, Ritalin can seem like a miraculous cure. But in the long term, it will cause 'down-regulation' so the child will need even more stimulation. This is probably why children given Ritalin are more likely to abuse other dopamine-promoting drugs and are more likely to become dependent on such drugs later in life.[149]

For these children, the stimulating brain nutrient DMAE (sold as Deanol in the US) is highly effective. Researcher and psychiatrist Dr Charles Grant discovered that in addition to increasing acetylcholine (the 'memory' neurotransmitter), in higher doses DMAE can actually block the acetylcholine receptor. This allows more dopamine to be released, thereby stimulating the brain. This action could explain DMAE's proven success with reward deficiency syndrome and ADHD.

Unlike Ritalin, DMAE doesn't increase the need for external stimulation and doesn't have all the undesirable side-effects.

So, for any child who has ADHD or hyperactivity, we recommend the following steps.

- Follow the guidelines in Part 1 regarding nutrients, sugar, essential fats and heavy metals.

- Eliminate chemical food additives and check other potential allergens such as wheat, dairy, chocolate, oranges and eggs.

- Consider supplementing DMAE under the guidance of your doctor or nutritional therapist.

CHAPTER 17

Moving Off the Autistic Spectrum

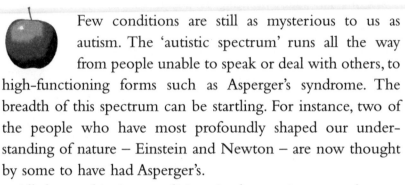Few conditions are still as mysterious to us as autism. The 'autistic spectrum' runs all the way from people unable to speak or deal with others, to high-functioning forms such as Asperger's syndrome. The breadth of this spectrum can be startling. For instance, two of the people who have most profoundly shaped our understanding of nature – Einstein and Newton – are now thought by some to have had Asperger's.

All the overlapping conditions in the previous two chapters – dyslexia, dyspraxia and ADHD – are often present in autism. For this reason, some are beginning to feel that this trio of conditions actually belongs in the autistic spectrum, as the highest-functioning forms. But autism is a distinct condition, with specific symptoms. These include difficulties with speech; abnormalities of posture or gesture; problems with understanding the feelings of others; sensory and visual misperceptions, fears and anxieties; and behavioural abnormalities such as compulsive/obsessive behaviour and ritualistic movements. Fits and convulsions are also common in severe autistics – see page 185 for a discussion of the condition and ways to combat it.

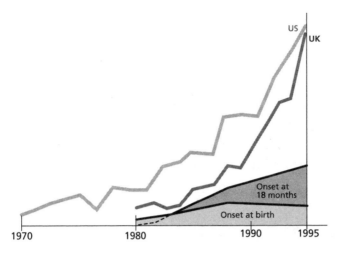

*This graph shows that autism is on the increase in the US and the UK;
The bottom right hand corner illustrates the change in relation to onset of
autism*

The US State Department of Developmental Services has
found that the incidence of autism more than tripled between
1987 and 1999.[150] The figures for the UK range from 3 to 10
times more cases over the last decade. While autism used to occur
primarily 'from birth', or at least was detected within the first 6
months, in both the US and UK over the past 10 years there has
a dramatic increase in 'late-onset' autism, most frequently diagnosed at age 2. According to the UK National Autistic Society,
the incidence may now be higher than 1 in every 100 children.

This strongly suggests that something new is triggering an
epidemic. Possible culprits include diet, vaccinations and
gastrointestinal problems, which are also very much on the
increase in children.

Six-year-old Andrew is a case in point. He had been diagnosed
with autism at age two and a half. He had frequent ear
infections and was a very picky eater, often restricting his diet
to two foods – chicken nuggets and chips. Tests revealed that he

had a number of food allergies and was low in magnesium. An analysis of his diet showed that he was taking in enormous amounts of sugar. Reducing sugar, supplementing magnesium and excluding the foods he was allergic to brought about some significant changes. Within a few weeks, his parents noticed and others began commenting that he seemed much brighter, more smiley and affectionate and had better eye contact. He ceased having ear infections and the range of foods that he would eat broadened considerably.

Unravelling autism

As with all conditions like this, there is the question as to whether it is 'inherited' or caused by something in diet or environment. Autism is four times as common in boys as girls. Parents and siblings of autistic children are far more likely to suffer from milk or gluten allergy, or have digestive disorders such as irritable bowel syndrome, high cholesterol, night blindness, light sensitivity, thyroid problems or cancer. Not being breastfed also increases the risk.

At first glance, it might seem that autistic children inherit certain imbalances. However, an alternative explanation might be that other family members have the same biochemical imbalances, eat the same food and may be lacking the same nutrients.

Given the overlap with dyslexia, dyspraxia and ADHD, all the factors discussed in the previous two chapters are also relevant in dealing with autism. So if your child is autistic, you'll need to help them balance blood sugar, check for brain-polluting heavy metals, exclude food additives, identify food allergies, correct digestive problems and possible nutrient deficiencies, and ensure an optimal intake of essential fats. There is growing evidence that these approaches can really make a big difference to children with autism. And that is certainly our experience at the Brain Bio Centre.

Nutrient deficiencies

We've known since the 1970s that a nutritional approach can help autism, thanks to the pioneering research by Dr Bernard Rimland of the Institute for Child Behaviour Research in San Diego, California. He showed that vitamin B6, C and magnesium supplements significantly improved symptoms in autistic children. In one of his early studies back in 1978, 12 out of 16 autistic children improved, then regressed when the vitamins were swapped for placebos.[151] In the decades following Dr Rimland's study, many other researchers have also reported positive results with this approach.[152]

Still others have, however, failed to confirm positive outcomes with certain nutrients. For example, a French study of 60 autistic children found they improved significantly on a combination of vitamin B6 and magnesium, but not when either nutrient was supplemented alone.[153] This study shows how important it is to get the balance of these nutrients right. It's likely to be different for each child.

B6 in particular may help, in part because many children with autism or learning difficulties have pyroluria, a condition in which, for genetic reasons, high levels of compounds called kryptopyrroles are excreted in the urine, causing a deficiency of zinc and vitamin B6. All children on the autistic spectrum should be screened for pyroluria. This involves a simple urine test (see Resources, page 279) and supplementing with appropriate levels of B6 and zinc, which have brought about remarkable improvements.

A lack of the right fats

Deficiencies in essential fats are common in people with autism.[154] Research by Dr Gordon Bell at Stirling University has shown that some autistic children have an enzymatic defect that removes essential fats from brain cell membranes more quickly than it should. This means that an autistic child is likely to need a higher intake of essential fats than the average. And it has been found that supplementing EPA, which can slow the activity of the defective enzyme, has clinically improved behaviour, mood, imagination, spontaneous speech, sleep patterns and focus of autistic children.[155-6]

The link with vitamin A

Paediatrician Mary Megson from Richmond, Virginia, believes that many autistic children are lacking in vitamin A. Otherwise known as retinol, vitamin A is essential for vision, as we've seen in this book. It is also vital for building healthy cells in the gut and brain. There is no real doubt that something funny is going on in the digestive tracts of autistic children. So how does vitamin A fit into the puzzle?

The best sources of vitamin A are breast milk, organ meats, milk fat, fish and cod liver oil, none of which are prevalent in our diets. Instead, we have formula milk, fortified food and multivitamins, many of which contain altered forms of retinol such as retinyl palmitate, which doesn't work as well as the fish- or animal-derived retinol. Megson began speculating what might happen if these children weren't getting enough natural vitamin A.[157]

She realised that not only would this affect the integrity of the digestive tract, potentially leading to allergies. It would also affect the development of their brains, and disturb their vision. Both brain differences and visual defects have been detected in autistic children. The visual defects, Megson deduced, were an important clue because lack of vitamin A would mean poor black-and-white vision, a symptom often seen in the relatives of autistic children.

If you can't see black and white, you can't see shadows. And without that you lose the ability to perceive three-dimensionality. This in turn leaves you less able to make sense of people's expressions, which could explain why some autistic children tend not to look straight at you. They look at you sideways. Long thought to be a sign of poor socialisation, this sideways technique may in fact be the best way for them to see people's expressions, because there are more black-and-white light receptors at the edge of the visual field than in the middle!

Of course, the proof is in the pudding. And Megson has reported rapid and dramatic improvements in autism simply by giving cod liver oil containing natural, unadulterated vitamin A. Often she has seen results within a week of starting children off on the oil.[158] Here are some of the comments her patients have made after cod liver supplementation. 'Now I know where my fingers are.' 'Now I can see my arms at the same time I see my fingers!' 'My box is getting bigger every day. Now I can see emotion on the faces on TV.'

We recommended cod liver oil supplementation for a seven-year-old with Asperger's. As his mother said, 'In the two weeks since following your advice there has been a significant improvement in his eye contact.' Although you need to be careful about the overall amounts of this fat-soluble vitamin your child takes (see page 132), vitamin A could be an avenue worth pursuing.

Allergies – undesirables on board

In addition to these likely deficiencies, the most significant contributing factor in autism appears to be undesirable foods and chemicals that often reach the brain via the bloodstream because of faulty digestion and absorption. Much of the impetus for recognising the importance of dietary intervention has come from parents who've noticed vast improvements in their children after changing their diets. As we've seen elsewhere in this book, certain foods and substances appear to adversely influence a large number of children, including:

- Wheat and other gluten-containing grains

- Milk and other dairy products containing casein

- Citrus fruits

- Chocolate

- Artificial food colourings

- Paracetamol

- Salicylates (see page 161).

The strongest direct evidence of foods linked to autism involves wheat and dairy, and the specific proteins they contain – namely, gluten and casein. These are difficult to digest and, especially if introduced too early in life, may result in an allergy. Fragments of these proteins, called peptides, can have big impacts in the brain. They can act directly in the brain by mimicking the body's own natural opioids (such as the enkephalins or endorphins), and so are sometimes called 'exorphins'. Or they can disable the enzymes that would break down these naturally occurring compounds.

In either case, the consequence is an increase in opioid activity, leading to many symptoms we describe as autism. Researchers at the Autism Research Unit at Sunderland University have found increased levels of these peptides in the blood and urine of children with autism.[159]

Gut feelings

To understand how these common foods can be so harmful to sensitive individuals, we need to look at how they get into the body via the gut.

As we saw above, exorphin peptides are derived from incompletely digested proteins, particularly food containing gluten and casein. One of these, called IAG and derived from gluten in wheat, has been detected in 80 per cent of autistic patients.[160] So the first problem is the poor digestion of proteins. A lack of sufficient zinc and vitamin B6 could contribute to this, as both are essential for proper stomach acid production and protein digestion, yet are often deficient in autistic children with pyroluria, as we saw above.

Whatever the case, however, partially digested protein fragments shouldn't be entering the bloodstream. So how do they? Vitamin A deficiency is certainly one culprit, but there may be more.

Many parents of autistic children report that their child received repeated or prolonged courses of antibiotic drugs for ear or other respiratory infections during their first year, before the diagnosis of autism. In Chapter 9, we saw how broad-spectrum antibiotics kill good as well as bad bacteria in the gut, weakening the intestinal membranes. This can lead to what is known as leaky gut syndrome, in which large molecules that shouldn't be absorbed through the gut membrane do get through.[161] And one kind of these could be exorphin peptides.

When Dr Andrew Wakefield of London's Royal Free Hospital studied 60 autistic children with gastrointestinal symptoms, he found many more intestinal lesions in them than in non-autistic children with similar digestive problems. In fact, over 90 per cent of the autistic children had chronically inflamed guts as a result of infection.[162]

So if your child has autism, restoring a healthy gut is vital. You can start simply, by supplementing digestive enzymes, and giving probiotics to restore the balance of gut bacteria. Both measures help heal the digestive tract and promote normal absorption, and have produced positive clinical results in autistic children.[163] Probiotics may also help your child digest exorphins before they can be absorbed.[164]

The amino acid L-glutamine helps to restore the integrity of the digestive tract. If you give 500mg dissolved in water to your child just before bedtime, this can be an effective way to help speed up gut healing and reduce allergic sensitivity. However, some autistic children have difficulty processing amino acids such as glutamine, which can result in the production of ammonia. Therefore we recommend seeking the guidance of a qualified nutritional thereapist first.

Cutting out wheat and dairy

Adding supplements to your child's diet is important, but so is removing any suspect food. There are many anecdotal reports of dramatic improvements in children with autism from parents who removed casein (milk protein) and gluten (the protein in wheat, barley, rye and oats) from their diet.[165] It can take some time for harmful peptides to leave the blood and brain, however, so results can be slow to emerge.

Dr Robert Cade, professor of medicine and physiology at the University of Florida, has observed that as levels of peptides in the blood decrease, the symptoms of autism decrease. 'If [levels of peptides] can be reduced to normal range,' he says, 'we typically see dramatic improvements.' (See graph, below.) But you need to help your child rigidly adhere to a strict gluten/casein-free diet to accomplish this.[166]

If you decide to go down this route with your child, you'll need to take a go-slow approach. The Autism Research Unit at Sun-

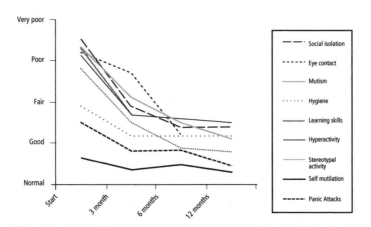

Symptom improvement observed in 70 autistic children while on a gluten/casein-free diet over twelve months

derland University recommends a gradual withdrawal of foods, waiting three weeks after the removal of dairy foods (casein) before removing wheat, oats, barley and rye (gluten) from the diet. Initially, your child may go through 'withdrawal' and their symptoms may get worse for a bit. Reducing slowly will help this.

Keep a food diary and note your child's behaviours and symptoms alongside all the foods they're eating. This can help to identify which of the usual suspects they are sensitive to – citrus fruits, chocolate, artificial food colourings, salicylates, eggs, tomatoes, avocados, aubergine, red peppers, soya and corn.[167] But remember, most of the foods in this list contain valuable nutrients, too, so you'll have to ensure that they are replaced rather than just removed. As you'll also need to be fully aware of which foods contain gluten and/or casein (see below), this entire process is best done under the guidance of a nutritional therapist (see Resources, page 274).

Tracking down gluten and casein

Grains containing gluten include wheat (and its species and hybrids, spelt, triticale and kamut), oats, barley and rye. That means you will need to cut out most bread, biscuits, cakes, pasta, breakfast cereals, bulghur, couscous, pizza, pitta bread, wraps, chapattis, naans, egg noodles, pastry, bagels, crumpets, pot noodles, pies, sausages, ready meals and processed foods. Check ingredient lists carefully and avoid any products containing flour, rusk, malted flake, modified starch or wheat starch. Most alternatives are based on rice or corn, and gluten-free breads, pastas, cereals, biscuits, crackers, cakes and bars are now readily available in health food shops and some supermarkets.

Casein is in all dairy products, including cow's milk, butter, cheese, yoghurt, ice cream and milk chocolate. Sometimes

---

goat's or sheep's milk are better tolerated, but you need to remove these from your child's diet too. Make use of the many soya alternatives now available – they include milk, cheese, yoghurt and ice cream. However, soya itself can also be a problem because some people develop sensitivity to it. So don't rely on it too heavily, and if you suspect your child has developed an intolerance to it, use alternatives made from rice and other gluten-free grains, which are also now widely available in health food shops.

Going for detox

Peptides can also harm the autistic child via the liver. This organ's job is that of a sophisticated cleaner's – detoxifying harmful chemicals and breaking down hormones and neurotransmitters.

Through a process called sulphation, the liver inactivates excess amounts of many neurotransmitters in the brain that modulate mood and behaviour, and so keeps the brain in balance. However, 95 per cent of autistic children have low sulphate levels, which may be inadequate for keeping levels of these neurotransmitters in check. Not only that: reduced sulphation also affects the mucin proteins that line the gastrointestinal tract, making the gut leakier and promoting inflammatory bowel disease. And this in turn allows peptides in, where they proceed to reduce sulphate production. It's a vicious circle.

The enzyme sulphite oxidase also plays a role in sulphate production, and levels of it are often low in autistic children. Sulphite oxidase is dependent on adequate levels of the mineral molybdenum, so supplementing this can be helpful – about 20 per cent of autistic children respond well to it.[168] Also potentially helpful in this context is a highly usable form of sulphur called MSM. For advice on dosage, we recommend you consult a qualified nutritional therapist.

Detoxification of the gut can also be helpful. Autistic children often have dysbiosis – the presence of undesirable microorganisms in the gut, whether bacteria, yeasts, fungi or parasites. Treatment with anti-fungal drugs such as Nystatin can get remarkable results, but note that children often get worse before they get better – fungi such as candida produce all sorts of toxins as they die off. Other less aggressive anti-fungal agents, including caprylic acid from coconut, charcoal and the yeast *Saccharomyces boulardii*, can be equally effective without triggering really severe reactions.

We strongly recommend you work with a nutritional therapist, who can advise you and your child on a suitable plan for detoxification, rather than doing it alone (see Resources, page 274, for details).

The big debate – MMR and autism

Does the MMR vaccine trigger autism? The issue has been hotly debated in the press, and among concerned parents in schoolyards across the UK. The official line is that there's no good evidence for any link between autism in children and the MMR. Of course, the last thing the medical profession want is a whole lot of children not being vaccinated, since that increases the risk of epidemics. But it is true that Dr Andrew Wakefield's research at the Royal Free Hospital,[169] while important, is only the first hint of a problem and it is probably too early to jump to conclusions.

It is, however, useful to look at what Wakefield actually said in this context:

Although MMR cannot by any means be described as a cause of autism, a child genetically predisposed to asthma, eczema, food allergy or intolerance, perhaps with possible disruption of the gut flora or with a fungal overgrowth, deficient in vitamins, minerals and essential fats, may be at risk from MMR. For them MMR could be described as the straw that broke the camel's back, tipping the balance of normal childhood development into a retrogressive state.[170]

For most children, the MMR vaccine is unlikely to be a problem, but having said this, no one really knows the full consequences of giving a child three immune attacks – mumps, measles and rubella – all at the same time. Getting all three illnesses at once simply doesn't occur in nature, so there's a logical argument for single vaccines if a parent so chooses, especially for children with weakened immune systems. Perhaps for children with nutrient deficiencies, a lack of essential fats, and a susceptibility to food allergies, infections and/or gut problems, these triple vaccines really *are* the last straw.

But is there any hard evidence against MMR? First, studies have shown a high incidence of autism in children whose mothers had received live virus vaccines (particularly the MMR or rubella vaccine) immediately before conception, or immediately following birth.[171] Secondly, there are two classifications of autism: one where autistic traits are noted from birth, and one where symptoms are noted at 18 months plus. The onset of autism at 18 months was uncommon until the mid-1980s, when the MMR vaccine came into wide use. After that, the incidence shot up.[172]

According to Dr Bernard Rimland of the Institute for Child Behaviour Research in San Diego, the problem may not be the vaccine itself, but a preservative used in multi-dose vials of many childhood vaccines till very recently. Thimerosal, a preservative containing high levels of mercury, was used in many vaccines up until 2001. Before this, each vaccine injection exposed the child to levels of toxic mercury in excess of the US federal government's own safety guidelines, and a child receiving all their jabs could have received a total of 187.5mcg of mercury – enough to give them heavy-metal poisoning.[173]

Mercury is known to inhibit the enzyme that digests gluten and casein, possibly increasing a child's susceptibility to wheat and milk allergy. Thus this heavy metal in vaccines may have the knock-on effect of contributing to the food allergies we frequently see in autism.

There's another fact that strengthens the link between autism and MMR. Many autistic children have been found to have measles antibodies in their gut. It's a bit like having a chronic infection, and seems to indicate that the triple vaccine makes measles persist. One of the most important allies the body has to fight off this virus is vitamin A – and Dr Megson's research (see page 174) indicates that many autistic children lack this key nutrient.

So, although it is too early to say yea or nay conclusively, it is entirely possible that late-onset autism may be triggered by multiple vaccinations, allergies, toxic overload or nutritional deficiencies – and especially combinations of any of these that send a child's gut and brain into distress.

A natural way with autism

It can be hard work, but the optimum nutrition approach to helping your autistic child is much more effective than the available drugs – and has no negative side-effects. It involves healing the digestive tract, avoiding sources of casein and gluten plus any other identified allergens, eating healthy foods, and supplementing nutrients that help support digestion, absorption, liver detoxification, the immune system and the brain.

As for drugs such as Ritalin, these are in any case generally not recommended for 'classic' autism, except when it is accompanied by ADHD or hyperactivity. In one survey of 8,700 parents asked to rate the effectiveness of drugs and other interventions, it was found that Ritalin was the most commonly prescribed – but only 26 per cent reported any improvement in their child, while 46 per cent said their child got worse on it. The most efficient drug in this survey, the anti-fungal Nystatin, was still found to help only 49 per cent of children taking it.[174]

As the story below of Habbo clearly shows, the optimum nutrition route can, by contrast, result in tremendous and lasting improvements. (This case study was kindly supplied by Emar Vogelaar from the European Laboratory of Nutrients in the Netherlands – see Resources, page 279, for further details.)

> Habbo was diagnosed as autistic at the age of four. He had serious speech and language problems, was severely behind in social and emotional development and attended special education for children with developmental delay. He had shown some improvement after taking special multivitamins, minerals and DMG (dimethyl glycine, a 'brain food') prior to visiting a clinic attached to the European Laboratory of Nutrients.
>
> Here Habbo was given comprehensive biochemical testing for deficiencies and imbalances. The clinic found low levels of five vitamins (A, beta-carotene, B3, B5 and biotin) and three minerals (magnesium, zinc and selenium). He also had low levels of omega-3 fats and the omega-6 fat GLA, as well as the amino acids taurine and carnitine. His digestion was poor, and he had abnormal gut flora and indications of a yeast infection. Food allergy testing showed a clear sensitivity to milk products and some other foods.
>
> He was given a special diet free from milk and casein, a personalised supplement programme, and later the anti-fungal drug Nystatin. He also started a programme of Applied Behaviour Analysis, working with a therapist.
>
> He improved steadily and was able to attend his local primary school from the age of six.

According to the Autism Research Institute's evaluation list, his improvements were:

Speech/language	from 36 to 89%
Sociability	from 13 to 68%
Sensory/cognitive awareness	from 22 to 97%
Health/physical behaviour	from 64 to 96%

(Where 100% means non-autistic behaviour)

By his fifth birthday, Habbo had had absolutely no interest in presents or visitors. One year after the evaluation, just before his eighth birthday, he made a list of eight presents he would like to have, including a computer. His parents told him the evening before to wake them at 7.30am on his birthday, and that's exactly what he did. During the day he couldn't wait for his friends to arrive and celebrate his special day.

Fits, convulsions and epilepsy

Profoundly autistic children may be prone to epilepsy. Although it's less common, people on the 'broader' autistic spectrum – including ADHD, dyslexia and dyspraxia – may also have fits or convulsions. Convulsions, which can last for seconds or minutes, are thought to be the result of a temporary upset in the brain's chemistry, causing neurons to fire off faster than usual and in bursts.

Neurological problems such as a brain injury, a stroke, an infection and, less frequently, a tumour can all bring on convulsions. High levels of stress and panic attacks can also trigger them, as can heart disease, especially irregular heartbeats, and blood sugar problems. Whatever the cause, convulsions indicate that the brain is out of balance, so an obvious place to start is to ensure an optimal intake of the brain's best friends – nutrients.

Many researchers have pointed out that people who have

convulsions or epilepsy are often deficient in certain nutrients – usually folic acid, the minerals manganese and magnesium, and essential fats.

Nutrients that counter convulsions

B vitamins Folic acid is depleted by convulsions, suggesting that it is somehow involved in them.[175] So it is ironic that anti-convulsant drugs such as phenytoin, primidone and phenobarbital further deplete folic acid.

Combining a drug such as phenytoin with folic acid works better than the drug alone. In one study, epileptics were given this drug with either folic acid or a placebo; after a year, only those on folic acid reported substantially fewer fits.[176] However, folic acid could be a double-edged sword. Some studies without control groups suggest that supplementation with this nutrient may actually cause epileptic fits in a minority of people. Several controlled studies, however, have failed to confirm this observation, suggesting that the incidence must be very rare.[177] With the guidance of your doctor, folic acid supplementation is well worth trying, although you can't expect immediate results.

Also worth supplementing is vitamin B6, which in high doses can produce almost immediate results. The first research to identify a role for B6 in the treatment of epilespy in children took place in Japan in the 1980s. More than half the children with 'infantile spasms' responded very well to B6 supplementation, although the doses used were very high and did cause side-effects in some participants.[178]

In a more recent study at the University of Heidelberg in Germany, 17 children were given high doses of vitamin B6 (300mg/kg/day). Five out of the 17 had immediate relief within two weeks, while after four weeks all of the patients were more or less free of seizures. No serious adverse reactions were noted. Side-effects were mainly gastrointestinal symptoms, and were reversible after the dosage was reduced.[179]

Magnesium, manganese and zinc The mineral manganese is essential for proper brain function and, to date, four studies have shown a correlation between low levels of it and epilepsy, suggesting that as many as one in three children with epilepsy have low manganese levels.[180-182]

In one study, published in the *Journal of the American Medical Association*, one child found to have half the normal blood manganese levels didn't respond to any medication, but on supplementing manganese had fewer seizures and improved speech and learning.[183] The late Dr Carl Pfeiffer, one of the pioneers of nutritional medicine, was the first to report the successful treatment of epilepsy with manganese.[184] At the Brain Bio Centre we have frequently found that patients with convulsions or fits are manganese deficient and have no or fewer fits once supplementation is begun. Manganese is found mainly in seeds, nuts and grains and tropical fruit such as bananas and pineapples. (Tea is very rich in it too, but we do not recommend children drink tea, as it's a stimulant.)

Magnesium is another mineral well worth checking out if your child is having fits or convulsions. Magnesium is vital for proper nerve and brain function, and, once again, a number of researchers have found low levels in patients with epilepsy and reported fewer fits on supplementation.[185-186] In animals, magnesium injections have also been shown to instantly suppress convulsions.[187]

If a child is found to have low blood levels of magnesium, as many as 75 per cent respond, with fewer fits, according to research from Romania.[188] Supplementing this mineral is especially helpful for those with 'temporal lobe' epilepsy, where a person has hallucinations of sound or smell, say, before a fit. This is hopeful news for children with this type of epilepsy, as they rarely respond to conventional anti-convulsant drugs.[189]

Finally, it's also well worth testing for zinc, as children with epilepsy can have lower levels of this mineral,[190] and anti-convulsant drugs can deplete it further. There is also data suggesting that having high levels of copper and a lack of zinc may increase the odds of having a seizure.[191] Ideally, we need to take in 10 times more zinc than copper. Zinc is also a valuable ally for vitamin B6, since it helps convert B6 (pyridoxine) into the active form of the vitamin, called pyridoxal-5-phosphate. It is highly likely that the few children who have had adverse reactions to very high doses of vitamin B6 may not have done so if given B6 together with zinc.

In fact, most adverse reactions to vitamins or minerals arise when they are treated like drugs and given at very high doses without other nutrients, thereby completely ignoring the principle of synergy – where nutrients working together amplify each others' action. For this reason, we strongly recommend that if your child is experiencing fits, convulsions or epilepsy, you see a nutritional therapist for a thorough nutritional workout.

This should involve both hair and blood analyses for magnesium, manganese and zinc, as well as folic acid. Levels of magnesium and folic acid are best tested in red blood cells. Depending on the results, a nutritional therapist can work out what combination of these nutrients, often in high doses, is worth trying, together with basic multivitamin supplementation.

An all-round good diet and supplements programme is, in fact, especially important, since other nutrients have also been shown to have positive effects on mental health in people with epilepsy. These include vitamin B1,[192] selenium[193] and vitamin E.[194] Some anti-epileptic medication depletes vitamin D, and some early research suggests that low levels of this vitamin may also contribute to seizures. If your child is taking anti-epileptic medication, get a blood test for vitamin D too.

Essential fats   One of the hottest areas of research into epilepsy is the effect of essential fat deficiency. So many people are deficient in omega-3s, in fact, that it's highly likely a significant proportion of people with epilepsy are also deficient; and there is intriguing evidence to show that supplementation can reduce the incidence of convulsions.

In one study, omega-3 and omega-6 essential fats, in a ratio of 1:4, were given to epileptic rats. After three weeks, up to 84 per cent fewer of the rats were having seizures, and the seizures that did occur tended to be very brief – there was up to a 97 per cent reduction in their duration. The team of researchers think this result was down to the positive effect of essential fats on stabilising signals between brain cells.[195]

Omega-3s also work in humans. Researchers at the Kalanit Institute for the Retarded Child in Israel gave children with epilepsy 3g of omega-3 fats for six months and found a dramatic reduction in both the number and severity of epileptic seizures.[196]

A word of caution in giving essential fat supplements to your epileptic child: we would advise you not to supplement omega-6s, as there is some evidence that this may increase seizures in children who have epilepsy.

Amino acids, phospholipids and herbs   Many of the 'brain food' nutrients discussed in Part 1, including phosphatidyl choline and essential fats, may also be helpful for children prone to fits. The brain's 'master tuners' – the amino acids SAMe and tri-methyl glycine (TMG) – are also potential aids (see also Chapter 14). A close relative of these, di-methyl glycine (DMG), produced remarkable results in one 22-year-old man with long-standing learning disabilities, who had been having around 17 seizures a week despite taking anticonvulsant medication. Within one week of starting 90mg of DMG twice a day, his seizures dropped to just three a week. When the DMG was withdrawn twice, the frequency of his seizures increased dramatically both times.[197]

The amino acid taurine, which helps to calm down the nervous system, may also help. In animals studies, low concentrations of taurine have been found in parts of the brain where seizure activity is highest, and supplementing taurine was found to have a potent, selective and long-lasting anticonvulsant effect.[198]

But the real star among these amino acids has got to be GABA, the brain's peacemaker, because it acts directly as a neurotransmitter. One possible mechanism for explaining why anticonvulsant drugs work is that they block the activity of the excitatory neurotransmitter, glutamic acid, and thereby promote the inhibitory neurotransmitter, GABA.

However, we would be cautious about supplementing GABA, and possibly large amounts of taurine, except under medical supervision. This is mainly because animal studies have shown that rats prone to petit mal seizures (where they seem 'absent' and stare blankly) sometimes have too much of these amino acids.[199] Another brain-friendly nutrient, DMAE, while potentially helpful, should also be given with caution. While DMAE is very helpful for many children with attention deficit disorder, a small percentage find it overstimulates; therefore, it should be used with caution, ideally under the guidance of a nutritional therapist, in children with manic tendencies or a history of epilepsy.

Vinpocetine, a herbal extract derived from the periwinkle plant (*Vinca minor*), may also help with fits, according to research in Russia.[200] This extract does many useful things in the brain, such as improving the production of cellular energy in neurons, and widening blood vessels so glucose and oxygen get to the brain more easily and are used more efficiently. As one theory about epileptic fits is that they're caused by fluctuations in glucose or oxygen supplies to the brain, this might explain why vinpocetine works.

So, the message here is that if your child is prone to fits, convulsions or epilepsy and hasn't been checked out by a nutritional therapist, there is plenty of room for hope.

If your child has autism, follow the nutritional strategy outlined here along with the recommendations at the end of Chapters 15 and 16.

- Eliminate gluten and dairy from your child's diet completely and replace them with the now readily available alternatives, while also checking the possibility of other food sensitivities under the guidance of a nutritional practitioner.

- Give your child cod liver oil, vitamin B6, magnesium, zinc, vitamin C, molybdenum, Saccharomyces boulardii and high-strength probiotics (minimum 4 billion microorganisms) daily.

- Ask your doctor to check your child for pyroluria and if they have it, include zinc and vitamin B6 in the above supplement regime.

- When considering the MMR vaccination, if your child has a weak immune system or you suspect nutrient deficiencies, low essential fats, susceptibility to food allergies, infections and/or gut problems, consider giving them single vaccines if they are available. Alternatively, address all of these issues with a nutritional therapist prior to their receiving the triple vaccine.

If your child has fits, convulsions or epilepsy, ensure you take the following steps. Note that as the recommended amounts of the supplements listed below depend on the age of your child, it is certainly best to see a nutritional therapist who can work out your child's ideal nutritional strategy.

- Balance your child's blood sugar and check for food allergies.

- Have his or her vitamin and mineral levels checked. If low in folic acid, B6, magnesium, manganese or zinc, supplementation may well help.

- Make sure he or she is getting enough essential fats, from seeds, fish and their oils.

- Other brain-friendly nutrients and herbs, including amino acids, phosphatidyl choline, DMAE, taurine and vinpocetine may help, but they are best taken under professional guidance.

CHAPTER 18

Answers for Aggression

 Has your child ever lashed out uncontrollably and violently towards you or someone else? It is a huge shock – and more, it can seem a complete mystery. But be assured that you are not alone. At the Brain Bio Centre, we see many cases of children, some very young, who are uncontrollable, violent and show no apparent remorse for their actions. Aggression in children is skyrocketing in the community, too. Sadly, the problem grows with the child, so as difficult as it may be when they are small, as they approach adulthood their future can look increasingly bleak.

But this scenario is in no way inevitable. You'll already have seen abundantly in this book how today's unbalanced, unhealthy diet affects the brain. And, true to form, we find that the major contributors to aggressive behaviour are the usual suspects – too much sugar, not enough essential fats, food allergies and brain pollution.

Eight-year-old Charles is a case in point. His parents brought him to see us at the Brain Bio Centre because they were concerned about his very aggressive and violent behaviour. Tests revealed food allergies, a homocysteine score of 14, and elevated aluminium in his hair. We recommended a specific supplement programmed designed to reduce homocysteine and to help his body detoxify the aluminium while also avoiding the foods that he was allergic to. After ten weeks, his parents reported that he was much more focussed, calmer and rational and wasn't lashing out like he had been. He had also stopped wetting himself, which had been a problem before.

As we have seen, all thoughts and consequently all behaviour are processed through the brain and nervous system, which are – like the rest of the body – completely dependent on nutrition to keep functioning. It's astonishing, but approximately half of all the glucose in the blood goes to power the brain, which is also dependent on a second-by-second supply of micronutrients – vitamins, minerals and essential fats. Meanwhile, any anti-nutrients in your child's body, such as lead and cadmium, will fundamentally affect brain function.

To date, there has been very little research into the effects of altering the diet of small children with aggression problems. However, there have been some excellent studies in adolescents, showing dramatic reductions in violent behaviour over a short space of time just by giving them small amounts of essential nutrients.

In one study at a young offenders' institution, the teenage inmates were given a multi-nutrient containing vitamins, minerals and essential fats, or a placebo. The results of this double-blind trial, published in the *British Journal of Psychiatry*, showed a staggering 35 per cent decrease in acts of aggression after only two weeks.[201] Common sense tells us that these nutrients would work even more effectively in small children before these behaviours have become a way of life.

Fighting back at aggressive behaviour

We feel there is much you can do to help your child nutritionally if they're often overcome with feelings of anger, or engage in aggressive behaviour. Let's look at some of the options.

Sorting out sugar-fuelled fury

The involvement of blood sugar fluctuations in behaviour is an intimate one. A 'rebound low', otherwise known as reactive hypoglycemia, can occur when a child consumes sugar, refined carbs or stimulants. The rapid rise in blood sugar levels can be followed by a crash, resulting in extreme tiredness, irritability, depression and aggression. And if a child feels this bad, they're much more likely to behave badly: exhaustion leads to poor impulse control.

If your child's behaviour is volatile and out of control, getting to grips with any blood sugar problems is vital. For more on how sugar affects your child's behaviour, and what to do to even that out, read Chapters 2 and 17.

Omegas – how to calm hostility

Recently, essential fats have increasingly been seen as a real contributor to aberrant behaviour. Changes in modern diets have certainly reduced our intake of these essential fats. And as we've seen, if the mother is deficient during pregnancy, it could have long-lasting effects on the child's mental development and behaviour.

Recent research from by Dr Tomohito Hamazaki of Toyama University in Japan suggests that omega-3 fats help control anger and hostility. He reasoned that under conditions of stress a certain level of aggression could have survival value, but from an evolutionary point of view, too much aggression would have the opposite effect.

So he decided to see what would happen to students under the stress of exams if given omega-3 fats. He gave them 1.5g of DHA, or a placebo, measuring hostility using psychological tests at the start of the study and again three months later, just before exams. The second test, just before the exams, showed a 59 per cent jump in hostile reactions in those taking the placebo, but no change at all in the students taking the omega-3 fats.[202] Omega-3 fats, it seems, help children to keep their heads under stress.

Countering nutritional deficiencies

Essential fats aren't the only key to calmer behaviour. Deficiencies in calcium, magnesium, zinc and selenium have all been shown to correlate with increases in violence.

The simple addition of a multivitamin and mineral supplement containing RDA levels of nutrients has been shown to have extremely positive effects on behaviour in prison populations in the US, according to extensive research by Dr Stephen Schoenthaler of the Department of Social and Criminal Justice at California State University, Stanislaus, whose work we looked at earlier.

In a recent study, Schoenthaler compared the behaviour of young offenders in the three months prior to and during supplementation, versus the behaviour of those given a placebo. There was an overall reduction in recorded offences of 40 per cent, with the subjects on supplements producing 22 per cent fewer assaults on staff and a 21 per cent reduction in violent and nonviolent antisocial behaviour compared with the subjects on placebo.

Blood tests for vitamins and minerals showed that around a third of the offenders had low levels of one or more vitamins and minerals before the trial. Those whose levels had become normal by the end of the study demonstrated a massive improvement in behaviour of between 70 and 90 per cent.[203] So it's not rocket science to make the leap that if adequate levels of these nutrients can have such dramatic effects on these adolescents, they will also help younger children with aggressive behaviour.

Antisocial foods

Severe allergic reactions can produce dramatic changes in behaviour, as has been well reported in hyperactive children with chemical or food intolerances[204] as well as in young offenders.[205] Read Chapter 9 for more information on brain allergies and how they may lead to seesawing moods.

Bipolar children

Some children with aggression problems have bipolar disorder – the condition formerly known as manic depression. They may oscillate from states of mania and hyperactivity to crying spells and depression. But the trouble is that bipolar disorder simply isn't diagnosed in childhood – in fact, it used to be thought that it didn't exist in the under-twenties. This is, however, a myth.

Bipolar disorder can and does occur in infancy, but the majority of these children are wrongly classified as having ADHD. Doctors Janet Wozniak and Joseph Biederman from Harvard Medical School found that 94 per cent of children with mania also met the criteria for a diagnosis of ADHD. This is bad news, because the last thing a child with bipolar disorder needs is stimulant drugs such as Ritalin.

Dr Demitri Papalos, associate professor of psychiatry at Albert Einstein College of Medicine in New York City, studied the effects of stimulant drugs on 73 children diagnosed as bipolar. Disturbingly, he found that 47 of these children were thrown into states of mania or psychosis by stimulant medication.[206] His excellent book, *The Bipolar Child*, co-authored with his wife Janice Papalos, helps to differentiate between children suffering from bipolar disorder and children with ADHD.

These are the characteristics and differences they've observed:

- Children with bipolar disorder essentially have a mood disorder and go from extreme highs, with mania, tantrums and anger, into extreme lows. Some may go through four cycles in a year, others in week-long cycles. This rapid cycling is rarely seen in adults.

- Bipolar children also have different kinds of angry outbursts. While most children will calm down in 20 to 30 minutes, bipolar children can rage on for hours, often with destructive, even sadistic, aggressiveness. They can also display disorganised thinking, language and body positions during an angry outburst.

- Bipolar children have bouts of depression, which is not a usual pattern of ADHD. Many show giftedness, perhaps in verbal or artistic skills, often early in life. Their misbehaviour is often more intentional, while the classic ADHD child often misbehaves through being inattentive. A bipolar child can, for example, be the bully in the playground.

The nutritional approach outlined below is likely to be helpful. Ritalin, and other stimulant drugs, can be an absolute disaster.

In summary, we recommend a number of steps for anyone whose child is aggressive or has violent mood swings.

- **Remove sugar and additives from their diet.**

- **Check for food allergies.**

- **See a nutritional therapist who can test your child for nutrient deficiencies as well as other biochemical imbalances which may be playing a part.**

- **Aggression is a psychological issue as well as a nutritional one, and you may find you need to follow a complementary approach. Alongside the methods suggested here, consider finding a therapist to address any psychological or family dynamic issues.**

CHAPTER 19

Overcoming Eating Disorders

 Anorexia and bulimia are complex and very serious conditions, and they are on the rise. But the good news is that they can be overcome.

If your child has recently become much thinner, how can you know whether they are simply undereating and losing weight, or have actually developed an eating disorder? First off, anorexia is very rare in under-12s, as is bulimia – a condition involving binge eating followed by self-induced vomiting and may involve overuse of laxatives. If your child is under 12, their thinness could be stemming from allergy, which would make the allergen foods a chore to cope with; or they may have developed a faddy attitude towards certain foods, perhaps egged on by their peers. (For help with food fads, see Chapter 22.)

But if your child is 12 or older, it is possible that they are showing anorexic tendencies. They may have been bullied about their weight at school, or unconsciously be trying to halt the physical changes of adolescence – and the inexorable progress towards adulthood – by controlling their body shape.

It's important to know what eating disorders 'look like', so you can take appropriate action when and if you need to. See the box below for signs you need to look out for.

What is an eating disorder?

Physical signs	Behavioural signs	Psychological signs
Anorexia nervosa	**Anorexia nervosa**	**Anorexia nervosa**
Severe weight loss	Wanting to be left	Intense fear of
Periods stopping	alone	gaining weight
(amenorrhoea)	Wearing big baggy	Depressed
Hormonal changes	clothes	Feeling emotional
in men and boys	Excessive	Obsession with
Difficulty sleeping	exercising	dieting
Dizziness	Lying about eating	Mood swings
Stomach pains	meals	Distorted
Constipation	Denying there is a	perception of body
Poor circulation and	problem	weight and size
feeling cold	Difficulty	
	concentrating	
	Wanting to have	
	control	
Bulimia	**Bulimia**	**Bulimia**
Sore throat/	Eating large	Feeling ashamed,
swollen glands	quantities of food	depressed and
Stomach pains	Being sick after	guilty
Mouth infections	eating	Feeling out of
Irregular periods	Being secretive	control
Dry or poor skin		Mood swings
Difficulty sleeping		
Sensitive or		
damaged teeth		
Binge eating	**Binge eating**	**Binge eating**
Weight gain	Eating large	Feeling depressed
	quantities of food	and out of control
	Eating inappropriate	Mood swings
	food	Emotional
	Being secretive	behaviour

Reproduced with permission of the Eating Disorders Association. Please see www.edauk.com for more details.

Missing the point

Anorexia was first identified by Dr William Gull in 1874. Sufferers eat often vanishingly small amounts of food in an attempt to suppress out-of-control feelings; they may also exercise obsessively. This was Gull's recommendation for treatment: 'The patient should be fed at regular intervals, and surrounded by persons who could have moral control over them, relations and friends being generally the worst attendants.'

Today's treatment is unfortunately not much different – summed up as 'drug them, feed them and let them get on with their lives' in an article in the *Guardian* describing treatment in 'leading hospitals'. This approach includes 'behaviour therapy' using rewards and privileges, and drugs to induce compliance. The drugs include psychotropic drugs such as chlorpromazine, sedatives and antidepressants. The diet is high-carbohydrate, sometimes as much as 5,000kcals, with little regard for quality.

Bulimia is probably the more common condition nowadays. Some anorexics are also bulimic, but not all bulimics are anorexic. Bulimia involves:

- Recurrent episodes of binge eating (rapid consumption of large amounts of food in a discrete period of time), at least twice a week

- A feeling of lack of control over eating during the binges

- Self-induced vomiting, use of laxatives, diuretics, strict dieting, fasting or exercise in order to prevent weight gain

- Persistent, obsessive concern with body shape and weight.

The underlying reasons for developing such severe and even life-threatening disorders can be many and tangled. Many people with anorexia or bulimia bear a secret, a trauma or a problem that needs to be resolved, and can be with the help and support of a psychotherapist.

But there are other possible strands to these difficult and puzzling conditions. Let's look at some of the latest research on nutritional links, which is leading to simple, pragmatic solutions that can work hand in hand with effective therapy.

The zinc link

The idea that nutrition, or malnutrition, could play a part in the development and treatment of anorexia did not really emerge until the 1970s and 1980s, when scientists began to realise just how similar the symptoms and risk factors of anorexia and zinc deficiency were. As early as 1973, researcher Michael Hambidge concluded that 'whenever there is appetite loss in children zinc deficiency should be suspected'.[207] In 1979, Rita Bakan, a Canadian health researcher, noticed that the symptoms of anorexia and zinc deficiency were similar in a number of respects, and proposed that clinical trials be undertaken to test the mineral's effectiveness in treatment.[208]

In fact, many risk factors in the two conditions are identical – both affect women under 25, and are linked to stress and puberty – as are many symptoms, including:

• Weight loss

• Loss of appetite

• Amenorrhoea (periods stopping)

• Impotence in males

• Nausea

• Skin lesions

• Malabsorption of nutrients

• Disperceptions

- Depression

- Anxiety.

Meanwhile, David Horrobin, most renowned for his research into evening primrose oil, proposed that 'anorexia nervosa is due to a combined deficiency of zinc and [essential fats]'.[209] More recently, strong evidence has come to light that those with anorexia and bulimia may be more prone to tryptophan deficiency. Tryptophan is the building block for serotonin, the brain's 'happy' neurotransmitter, which also helps control appetite.

Confirming the connection

In 1980, the first trial studying zinc and anorexia started at the University of Kentucky in the US. The researchers discovered that 10 out of 13 patients admitted with anorexia and 8 out of 14 patients with bulimia were zinc deficient on admission. Yet, after ample feeding, they became even more zinc deficient. Since zinc is needed for the digestion and utilisation of protein, from which body tissue is made, they recommended that extra zinc, above the amounts that would correct a deficiency, should be given as the anorexic starts to eat and gain weight.[210]

In 1984, the penny well and truly dropped with two important research findings. The first study, since confirmed, showed that animals deprived of zinc very rapidly developed anorexic behaviour and loss of appetite, and that if these animals were force-fed a zinc-deficient diet to gain weight, they became seriously ill.[211] The second study showed that zinc deficiency damages the intestinal wall and therefore the absorption of nutrients including zinc, potentially leading to a vicious spiral of deficiency.[212]

That same year, Professor Derek Bryce-Smith, now patron of the Institute for Optimum Nutrition, reported the first case of anorexia treated with zinc. The patient was a 13-year-old girl, tearful and depressed, weighing just 37kg. She was referred to a consultant psychiatrist, but despite counselling, three months later her weight was 31.5kg (under 5 stone). Then she began a course of zinc supplementation – 45mg a day. Within two months, she weighed 44.5kg and was cheerful again, and testing normal for zinc levels.[213]

In the mid-1980s meanwhile, the first double-blind trial with 15 anorexics began at the University of California. In 1987 the researchers reported: 'Zinc supplementation was followed by a decrease in depression and anxiety. Our data suggest that individuals with anorexia nervosa may be at risk for zinc deficiency and may respond favourably after zinc supplementation.'[214] By 1990, many researchers had found that over half of anorexic patients showed clear biochemical evidence of zinc deficiency.[215]

Zinc supplementation couldn't be easier, but sadly, many treatment centres still fail to offer it.

Chicken or egg?

The evidence linking zinc and anorexia is now beyond question. In fact, a recent review of all the research so far concludes: 'There is evidence that suggests zinc deficiency may be intimately involved with anorexia in humans: if not as an initiating cause, then as an accelerating or exacerbating factor that may deepen the pathology of anorexia.'[216]

But the fact that high levels of zinc supplementation help to treat anorexia does not mean that the cause of anorexia is zinc deficiency. It is psychological issues that usually trigger changes in the eating habits of susceptible people.

As mentioned above, anorexia can be a way of staving off adulthood and what are perceived as overwhelming fears and responsibilities. By avoiding eating, a young girl can repress the signs of growing up. Menstruation stops, breast size decreases and the body stays small. Starvation also induces a kind of 'high' by stimulating changes in important brain chemicals that may help to block out difficult feelings and issues that are too hard to face.

So where does zinc come in? Many anorexics choose to become vegetarian, and most vegetarian diets are lower in zinc, essential fats and protein, according to a study at the Health Sciences Department of the British Columbia Institute of Technology in Burnaby, Canada, which analysed the diets of vegetarian anorexics, versus non-vegetarian patients.[217]

Whether vegetarian or not, once the pattern of not eating is chosen and becomes established, zinc deficiency is almost inevitable, due both to poor intake and poor absorption. With it comes a further loss of appetite and even more depression and disperceptions, along with an inability to cope with the stresses that face many adolescents growing up in the 21st century.

The optimum nutrition approach to helping someone with anorexia or bulimia is best adopted alongside sessions with a skilled psychotherapist. The nutritional approach emphasises quality of food rather than quantity, including supplements to ensure vitamin and mineral sufficiency – including 45mg of elemental zinc a day, and half that once weight gain is achieved and maintained.

Tryptophan and appetite

A loss of weight and of muscle tissue indicates protein deficiency. Obviously, with anorexia or bulimia, the sufferer will not be getting enough protein, or they may be having trouble digesting, absorbing or metabolising it. The amino acids valine, isoleucine and tryptophan have been found to be low in people with anorexia. Supplementing valine and isoleucine helps to build muscle, while tryptophan is the building block of serotonin, which controls both mood and appetite.

Recent research has found striking differences in the blood levels of tryptophan in people with anorexia.[218] Both starvation and excessive exercise have emerged as factors in these levels.[219] So far, the evidence points to problems with how anorexics or bulimics respond to low levels of tryptophan. As the conversion of tryptophan into serotonin is both zinc and B6 dependent, all three nutrients may be needed for proper appetite control, as well as a balanced, happy mood.

The interplay between body and mind, or nutrients and behaviour, is well illustrated by recent research at Oxford University's psychiatry department by Dr Philip Cowen and colleagues. Cowen and his team found, not surprisingly, that levels of tryptophan and serotonin were lower in women on calorie-restricted diets. They also found, however, that recovered bulimics put on a diet free of tryptophan rapidly become more depressed and overly concerned about their weight and shape, as well as more fearful of losing control over their eating.[220]

Looked at together, all this research strongly suggests that people prone to anorexia or bulimia have a special need for tryptophan, and probably zinc and B6, and that when deprived of these nutrients they are more likely to develop unhealthy responses to stress, such as the loss of appetite control.

The most direct way of addressing these imbalances in people with eating disorders is to supplement tryptophan, or 5-hydroxytryptophan (5-HTP), plus zinc and B6. But in the long run, the goal has got to be a change in diet. Often, especially in anorexics, supplements such as concentrated fish oils are easier to handle at the start because, unlike food, they contain virtually no calories. As the person's nutritional status improves, their anxieties and obsessive/compulsive tendencies will ease off, and they will almost always see the logic of making positive dietary changes.

The ideal diet should include foods that are easy to eat

and digest as well as highly nutritious. Good-quality protein such as quinoa, fish, soya and spirulina or blue-green algae is important, as are ground seeds, lentils, beans, fruits and vegetables.

Fish and seeds are especially important because they contain essential fats. Since most people with eating disorders go out of their way to avoid fat, their diets are frequently low in these essential nutrients, which as we've seen really are essential when it comes to mental health. Also, essential fats are vital for both making serotonin and receiving the serotonin signals that cross from one neuron to another – spreading the happiness around, in effect.

Pinning down binge foods

The foods people with bulimia binge on are highly revealing, either of food sensitivities or blood sugar problems. The most common binge foods are sweet, wheat-based or dairy products. Both wheat and dairy products contain exorphins, chemicals that mimic (and can therefore block) pleasure-giving endorphins in the brain, and so possibly influence behaviour. And when the person's blood sugar is very low – as it would be after a fast or after vomiting – they would inevitably crave sweet foods for a quick sugar fix.

The effects of all these foods can contribute to the confusions and erratic or compulsive behaviour of people struggling with bulimia. We often ask people with bulimia to binge as much as they like for the next two weeks, but not on any of these foods. Many of them report that their desire to binge at all is dramatically reduced right away.

Don't think, however, that if your child is, say, more prone to react strongly to the lack of a nutrient like zinc or tryptophan, that that's the whole story. As we have said, biochemistry does not exclude psychological problems as part of the reason your child has developed an eating disorder. Seek constructive help from a sensitive and reliable therapist.

We have a number of recommendations for anyone who is dealing with an eating disorder.

- See a nutritional therapist who can assess what your child is deficient in and advise you accordingly.

- Their advice will probably include zinc, B6, 5-HTP, plus essential fats, either in capsules or in seeds and fish.

- Take your child to see a psychotherapist with experience of helping children with eating disorders make a full recovery.

CHAPTER 20

Curing Sleep Problems

 Can't sleep, won't sleep? Children's sleep problems are some of the most common parents face. The result isn't just mentally exhausted children who struggle to learn, concentrate and behave, but parents in a permanent state of tiredness themselves. Research showed many years ago that one key to growth and development in children is a good night's sleep – and that includes the growth and development of the brain.

So poor sleep delivers a double whammy: a short-term impact on your child's performance, energy and mood today, and an insidious curb on their development that prevents them from reaching their full potential as an older child and adult.

Seven-year-old James is a case in point. His mother brought him to see us at the Brain Bio Centre because, no matter how tired he became, he simply was not sleeping. Consequently he had terrible concentration and memory at school. We screened him for various biochemical imbalances and analysed his diet. We found that James had food allergies, low levels of calcium and magnesium and too much sugar in his diet. By excluding the foods that James was allergic to, reducing his sugar intake and supplementing extra calcium and magnesium, James's sleep improved significantly within a matter of weeks.

Is your child sleep-deprived?

Without sleep, even for a night, the body shows clear signs of stress – mood and concentration go, defences drop, zinc and magnesium levels fall, and vitamin C is used up at an alarming rate. Sleep rejuvenates both body and mind. In fact, during the first three hours of sleep, the body goes into rapid repair mode.

Sleep specialists at Loughborough University in the UK have carried out a series of tests into how the brain functions when it is deprived of sleep. And the results are very clear: sleepy people have problems finding the right words, coming up with ideas and coping with rapidly changing situations.[221] Sleep deprivation makes us moody and irritable, and in the long term, even depressed. Scientists have measured the body's ability to fight off infections when it is tired, and research has shown that sleep-deprived individuals have fewer natural killer cells, a type of immune cell needed for resistance against invaders.[222]

School-aged children need somewhere between 9 and 12 hours of sleep at night. But it's easy to tell if they're getting enough: they go to bed, fall asleep easily, wake up easily, and are not tired during the day.

There are two main types of sleep problems – trouble getting to sleep and trouble staying asleep. If your child resists going to bed and kicks up a fuss every night at bedtime, it could be that he or she faces the inevitable prospect of lying awake for hours feeling bored and frustrated before they finally drop off. And a television, games console or computer in the bedroom is not the answer, since research shows that these make sleep problems worse.

Judith Owens of the Brown University School of Medicine, Rhode Island, studied 495 children in kindergarten and primary school to determine what effect watching TV might have on their sleep patterns. She found that TV watching at bedtime, especially when the set was in the child's bedroom, was the strongest predictor of a bad night's sleep, with children taking longer to get to sleep and more likely to wake in the night.[223]

Finding the zzzzz factor

Whichever type of sleep problem is affecting your child, however, the factors to consider are the same: along with habitual telly-gazing last thing at night, these include deficiencies of the calming minerals magnesium and calcium, excess sugar or stimulants, food allergies and a lack of physical activity during the day.

Chill-out minerals

If your child fails to get enough magnesium and calcium, it can trigger or exacerbate sleep difficulties because this mineral duo work together to calm the body and help relax nerves and muscles. As we've seen, magnesium deficiency is increasingly common in children.

In fact, your child's diet is likely to be lower in magnesium than in calcium, so make sure they're eating plenty of magnesium-rich foods – seeds, nuts, green vegetables, wholegrains and seafood. Including some magnesium in the evening, perhaps even in a supplement, may help. If your breastfed baby is having trouble sleeping, you can take a magnesium supplement yourself and your baby will receive it through your milk. Particularly good sources of calcium, meanwhile, include milk products, green vegetables, nuts, seafood and molasses.

Other nutrients that are important for good sleep are the B vitamins. These are best taken earlier in the day rather than in the evening, though, as they are also involved in energy production and can be overstimulating just before bed.

Cutting out stress, sugar and stimulants

Many of the daily rhythms in your child's body, including those dictating energy and sleepiness, are finely tuned mechanisms that depend on certain hormonal patterns, chemicals and nutrients. At night, the levels of the stress hormone cortisol should dip, calming them down and preparing the body for sleep. If, however, their cortisol levels are out of kilter for any reason (usually stress or a diet high in stimulants or sugar), their ability to get to sleep, to sleep through the night or to wake up refreshed are likely to be impaired.

If cortisol levels are high at night, for instance, this suppresses the release of growth hormone, which is essential for daily tissue repair and growth. So it's an excellent idea to establish a 20- to 30-minute nightly 'calm-down' bedtime routine, which can include taking a bath, putting on pajamas, reading and other relaxing activities.

Many parents whose children wake in the night and then can't get back to sleep find that once they start keeping their blood sugar levels even during the day, that sets the scene for the correct patterns at night, giving them more chance of a good night's sleep. A light, low-GL snack half an hour to an hour before bed ensures not only that your child is not kept awake by hunger pangs, but also that he or she won't be woken during the night by a drop in blood sugar levels. A small piece of fruit and a handful of seeds or some nut butter on one or two oatcakes is ideal. Caffeine – and this includes chocolate – should be avoided entirely. Even small amounts taken early in the day can keep children awake at night.

Solving sleep apnoea

Children who have a chronically blocked nose may suffer from sleep apnoea, a condition usually associated with older adults. In sleep apnoea, your sleeping child will struggle to breathe to the point of waking up, or at least will have a very restless night.

If your child has a stuffy or runny nose and is a 'mouth-breather', you should suspect food allergies.

Read Chapter 9 for details on identifying and eradicating food allergies. Addressing food allergies can also be the answer for other sleep-associated problems such as bedwetting.

Serotonin and melatonin

The amounts of serotonin and the hormone melatonin in our bodies increase in the evening as part of our natural sleep–wake cycle. Deficiencies in either can prevent sleep, and disruptions in sleep patterns can deplete the body of these substances. The body needs adequate amounts of B6 and tryptophan to make serotonin and melatonin.

Foods particularly high in tryptophan are chicken, cheese, tuna, tofu, eggs, nuts, seeds and milk. So, as so often happens, a traditional remedy – drinking a glass of milk before bed – has become grounded in science. (Other foods associated with inducing sleep are lettuce, which contains a substance related to opium, and oats.)

5-HTP is the amino acid our bodies use to make serotonin and melatonin, so supplementing 5-HTP for a month can be useful as a way of normalising sleep patterns, once all the other obstacles to sleep have been addressed. When your child is sleeping well again, they can stop taking the supplements. We recommend 25mg an hour before bed for children under eight, and 50mg for older children.

Melatonin production in the body is lowered by light, so make sure all the lights in your child's bedroom are dimmed before they go to bed. Complete darkness is best for sleep. You can get up to 50mcg of melatonin, a tenth of 1mg (an adult supplement dose is between 1mg and 10mg daily), in a 3oz serving of oats, brown rice or sweetcorn. Bananas and tomatoes have half this amount. So serving these foods in the evening may help your child sleep.

Melatonin is a neurotransmitter, not a nutrient, and hence needs to be used much more cautiously when supplementing. Taking too much can cause diarrhoea, constipation, nausea, dizziness, headaches, depression and nightmares. However, melatonin has been used to good effect in children in a number of studies,[224–225] so is worth a try under the guidance of a qualified nutritional therapist or doctor. Melatonin cannot be bought over the counter in Britain, but is available by mail order or on the web from the US where these restrictions don't apply (see Resources, page 280).

Running out the restlessness

Ever watched your child tearing around a playground and thought, 'They'll sleep well tonight'? It's true: exercise de-stresses and promotes calmness and a sense of well-being, partly through the release of endorphins. So aside from PE at school, encourage your child to get active at weekends and in the afternoon rather than simply slumping in front of the TV or computer. They're sure to find something they enjoy: swimming, football with friends, tennis, dance class, or just a brisk walk in the park or a spin on their bike. Just ensure they don't exercise too late in the evening, as the energising effects of all that activity may promote sleeplessness.

To ensure your child get a good night's sleep, follow these sensible suggestions.

- **Avoid sugar and stimulants, especially after 4pm.**

- **Follow a regular, calming bedtime routine every evening.**

- **Supplement magnesium and calcium in the evening and ensure your child eats plenty of magnesium and calcium-rich foods such as seeds and crunchy or dark green vegetables.**

- To re-establish a good sleep pattern, try 10 to 25mg of 5-HTP and perhaps melatonin under supervision.

- Limit television to no more than 2 hours a day, and if there is a television, computer or games console in your child's bedroom, remove it.

- Ensure your child has plenty of stimulating physical activity during the day so they are ready for sleep in the evening.

PART 4

Food for Thought

Now that you know what optimum nutrition for your child's mind really means, how do put this into action? In this part we'll show you what to do to feed your child properly, from infancy to teenage years. You'll find masses of shopping tips, meal ideas and practical ways to keep your child's diet on track and choose the right supplements.

CHAPTER 21

Getting off to a Good Start

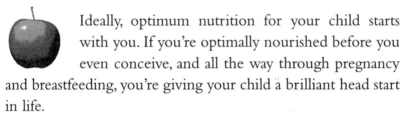 Ideally, optimum nutrition for your child starts with you. If you're optimally nourished before you even conceive, and all the way through pregnancy and breastfeeding, you're giving your child a brilliant head start in life.

Breast milk is, in fact, your child's optimum food for robust physical and mental health during those crucial first few months. Developing good food habits starts with the weaning process, when your two main objectives need to be keeping your child from developing food allergies, and ensuring they develop a taste for a wide range of healthy foods.

The smart way to feed your baby

As a way of nourishing your baby, breastfeeding is better by design. And not just for their physical development: breastfed babies are not only healthier all round and less prone to allergies in later life,[226] they are also smarter! A recent series of worldwide studies indicate that breastfed babies have an IQ 6 to 10 points higher than that of formula-fed babies.[227]

One reason for this is probably the high levels of the omega-

3 fat DHA that's found naturally in breast milk. As we've seen, DHA is vital for brain development. And the longer a baby is breastfed, the higher the intelligence they can expect to have as young adults.[228] Another reason for the higher intelligence is likely to be that the fat-soluble vitamins in breast milk are more easily absorbed.

In a Brazilian study, only one in 176 breastfed babies had lower than adequate levels of vitamin E, compared to more than half in a cow's milk formula-fed group.[229] Another study has shown that breast milk is higher in vitamin D than formula milk – and not just any vitamin D, but a particular kind which has been found to be 2.5 times more effective at preventing rickets – the deficiency disease where bones don't develop properly, which amazingly is on the increase in Britain.[230] There are also more brain-boosting minerals in breast milk than in most formulas. [231]

Breastfeeding also helps to establish healthy gut bacteria. A type of beneficial gut bacteria called bifidobacteria, present in breast but not formula milk, prevents harmful bacteria from invading your baby's gut. This is an important service, as it not only protects against colic, eczema and asthma, but crucially, as we saw in Chapter 9, also helps to prevent food allergies, which can affect the brain.

Breastfed babies are also less likely to be obese. A study of 32,000 Scottish children three to four years old found that those breastfed for six to eight weeks after birth were 30 per cent less likely to be obese than bottlefed children.[232] As the quality of your milk while breastfeeding is determined to a large extent by the quality of your diet, you'll need to be optimally nourished yourself, and also avoid any foods you might be allergic to since you can pass on food allergies through breast milk. (For more information on healthy nutrition during pregnancy and breast-feeding, read *Optimum Nutrition Before During and After Pregnancy* by Patrick Holford and Susannah Lawson.)

Keeping your child allergy-free

As with so much else, prevention is better than cure when it comes to allergies and your child. Preventing an allergy from developing in your child is much easier and better than trying to 'cure' them later. There are two important points here. One is the choice and timing of first foods, the other the health of your baby's digestive system.

First foods

Don't start weaning your child onto food earlier than you need to – start at around six months. It's preferable to breastfeed your baby exclusively up to this point. If they are failing to thrive on breast milk alone, visit your paediatrician and a nutritional therapist for advice before deciding to add other foods to their diet. A lack of solid foods or formula milk may not be the problem, and adding these to their diet may make things worse if poor digestion is an issue.

Since, as we saw in Chapter 9, some foods are more likely to cause allergies than others, a strategic introduction of the least allergenic foods into your baby's diet while their digestive tract is still immature is essential.

What and when to introduce while weaning

From 6 months
- Vegetables *except* tomatoes, potatoes, peppers and aubergines (members of the 'deadly nightshade' family)
- Fruits *except* citrus
- Pulses and beans
- Rice, quinoa, millet and buckwheat
- Fish (preferably organic, wild or deep sea)

From 9 months
- Meat and poultry (preferably organic)

- Oats, corn, barley and rye
- Live yoghurt
- Tomatoes, potatoes, peppers and aubergines
- Eggs
- Soya (as in tofu or soya milk)

From 12 months

- Citrus fruits
- Wheat
- Dairy products
- Nuts and seeds (but not peanuts – wait as long as you can before introducing these, and then, use only organic varieties)

It's a good idea to start a weaning diary so you can keep track of how your baby takes to the various foods you introduce. To begin with, introduce only one food each day, make a note of it and watch for any possible reaction. This could be anything from a skin rash or eczema, excessive sleepiness, a runny nose, an ear infection, dark circles under the eyes, excessive thirst, over-activity or asthmatic breathing. If you notice anything amiss, stop giving that food and then introduce another once the reaction has died down. You can double-check your observations by reintroducing these foods a few months later. By that time, your baby's digestive system will have matured, so they may no longer react to that food.

Once your baby is eating a mixture of foods that cause no reaction, it's then important to vary their diet as much as possible, especially with common allergenic culprits such as wheat, dairy, soya and citrus fruits. Eating the same thing over and over again long term can overtax the system and induce an allergy. But a varied diet will also boost your child's desire for a wider range of foods – and this will in turn ensure they're getting a broader range of nutrients.

Digestive health

Food allergies are intimately linked to poor digestive health – one seems to exacerbate the other. But keeping your baby's gut healthy is vital for a lot of other reasons, too.

For instance, gut and brain are closely connected via the nervous system – so closely that the gut is actually thought of as a second brain. Called the enteric nervous system, this network of neurons, neurotransmitters and proteins lining the gut is in constant communication with the central nervous system up in your brain and spinal cord. So keeping your child's gut healthy is also essential for optimising their brain development.

Unfortunately, many babies these days seem to have their first dose of antibiotics within days or weeks of birth, resulting in gastric upsets and more. Antibiotics wipe out the beneficial gut flora in the digestive tract, causing an imbalance in them that can in turn lead to food allergies, digestive problems and lower levels of essential minerals.[233] Links have even been found to ADHD.[234]

Antibiotics are usually given to babies for ear, nose and throat infections, which may themselves be caused by food allergies, particularly if they are recurrent. So it is well worth getting to the root of the problem and resolving food allergies. According to a study published in the *Journal of the American Medical Association*, antibiotics given for ear infections in children triples the chance of a repeat infection![235]

While breast milk contains beneficial gut flora that will recolonise your baby's gut following antibiotics, formula milk typically doesn't. If it's essential for your baby to take antibiotics, make sure you follow them with an age-appropriate probiotic supplement that will supply the right strains of gut flora. See Resources, page 281.

A good diet from the start

Once your child is onto solids, the next 18 months are absolutely crucial to establishing healthy eating. The emphasis should be on vitamin- and mineral-rich vegetables and fruit. Choose organic if you can, so you are not polluting your baby with residues from artificial fertilisers, herbicides or pesticides.

Many parents make the mistake of weaning their child onto a lot of fruit and 'baby cereals', both of which are very sweet. If you do this, you may find your child rejecting vegetables. So really prioritise vegetables over fruit. The less sweet food and drink your baby has, the less he or she will desire it. Also, remember that while you are spoon-feeding pureed broccoli into your baby's mouth, they're watching your facial expression. So look like you enjoy eating it too! It's very easy to unconsciously let your face screw up into a grimace while cooing 'Mmmm yummm' to your baby. He or she won't be fooled if your *face* is saying 'Ooh yuck!'

Make sure, too, that there's plenty of colourful variety. Dr Gillian Harris, a clinical psychologist at Birmingham University in the UK, has studied the impact of first foods on a child's food preferences later on. She found that babies weaned on rusks, baby food, processed foods and milk are more likely to go on to prefer 'beige carbohydrates' such as crisps, white bread and chips rather than eating their greens. Babies exposed to fruit, vegetables and a range of other 'non-beige' foods will, by contrast, show a greater preference for many-hued, nutrient-laden foods later on.

Dr Harris puts this down to an ancient survival mechanism. She believes that children build up a 'visual prototype' of favoured foods. This model meshes with evolutionary theory, which suggests that our tastes and preferences were shaped to help us survive.

We are born with a love of sweet tastes, associated with ripe fruit and breast milk, and a dislike of bitter tastes, linked for obvious survival reasons with alkaloid toxins in plants. But we can learn to change these tastes depending on what our parents give us to eat. However, at the age of around 18 months, when a Stone Age toddler would have been able to wander around and select their own food for the first time, the visual proto-type mechanism is turned on to prevent them from wanting to eat unfamiliar and potentially poisonous foods.

Does my child need to drink milk?

For as long as you breastfeed, you don't need to supplement your baby's diet with cow's milk. However, once you stop, you will need to ensure they get a good source of calcium. Milk has been marketed for decades as the perfect calcium-rich food, especially for young children. But the key word here is 'marketed'.

Early humans drank no milk after weaning – yet they still managed to develop strong bones and teeth. There is no evidence that once they ceased to be nomadic hunter-gathers and began to cultivate the land, eating grains and keeping animals for meat and milk, their bones got stronger. In fact, the opposite seems to be true. We appear to have shrunk in height by five or six inches! This, however, is thought to be due to difficulties in dealing with grain, more than to any problem with milk.[236]

We need to remember that milk is a specialised food full of hormones geared for calves, rather than us. And as we've seen, milk protein or casein causes digestive problems in a lot of people. Meanwhile, if it is so essential, where do the Chinese (for instance), whose consumption of milk is vanishingly small, get their calcium? From vegetables, nuts, seeds and soya prod-ucts. So while it's widely consumed by our society, milk doesn't seem to stand up as an essential for good health. And as many people develop allergies to it, it's not a good idea for your child to become too reliant on milk – as long as you make sure their diet is rich in other sources of calcium. See the table below for the best calcium-rich foods, which are important inclusions in your child's diet if they're avoiding dairy products.

If you decide you do want to give your child milk, reduce its allergic potential by rotating cow's milk with goat's and sheep's milks, plus soya, rice and nut milks (although you need to wait until they are a year old before introducing any nut products) – visit your local health food shop to find a full selection. We ourselves buy a variety and switch between them, using up one carton before starting on a different type of milk.

Yoghurt is often better tolerated than milk, as the live bacteria that make it predigest a lot of the problematic milk sugars and proteins. Live yoghurt, especially, where those bacteria remain intact, can help to promote a healthy digestive system. And the calcium in yoghurt is easier to absorb than that in milk. Goat's and sheep's yoghurt is easy to find these days, allowing you more variety.

Calcium in foods – the richest sources

per 100g/100ml	Calcium content (mg)
Cheddar cheese	720
Tahini (sesame seed paste)	680
Sesame seeds	670
Sardines canned in oil	550
Almonds	240
Spring greens, raw	210
Watercress	170
Brazil nuts	170
Kale	150
Tofu (enriched with calcium)	150
Blackstrap molasses (per tablespoon)	150
Whole milk	115

To get your child off to the best start in life, follow these rules.

- Breastfeed exclusively for at least four and preferably six months, then wean them following the guidelines in this chapter.

- During weaning, introduce plenty of colourful pureed vegetables rather than bland, sweet fruit or cereal mixes. And as you demonstrate eating it to your baby, look like you're enjoying it too!

- If your baby is given antibiotics, follow them with age-appropriate probiotics to replenish the beneficial gut flora. Seek advice from a nutritional therapist.

CHAPTER 22

Preventing Food Fads and Fussiness

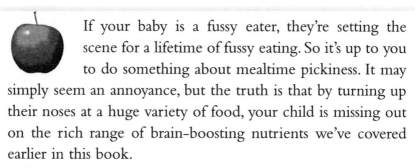 If your baby is a fussy eater, they're setting the scene for a lifetime of fussy eating. So it's up to you to do something about mealtime pickiness. It may simply seem an annoyance, but the truth is that by turning up their noses at a huge variety of food, your child is missing out on the rich range of brain-boosting nutrients we've covered earlier in this book.

You need to start early to ensure that your child actively enjoys eating a broad variety of healthy foods. If you leave it until they're older, the nay-saying will become more and more ingrained – and they will in any case listen to you less and less as they approach their teen years!

'My child will only eat...'

Which is it? Chocolate yoghurt? Spaghetti hoops? Baked beans? Potatoes, carrots and sausages? If you haven't said, 'My child will only eat...' yourself, you'll have heard it in the schoolyard or down the phone line from a desperate fellow parent. If you have missed the window of opportunity in your child's infancy to nip their fussy-eating tendencies in the bud (see Chapter 21), all is not lost – but now is the time to act.

First, go through your cupboards and fridge. If you don't actually store baked beans or sugary yoghurts, fizzy drinks or whatever other junk food your child says they want to eat, you have the perfect answer to their request: there isn't any. Meanwhile, you can be stocking up on healthy alternatives to the foods they like.

For homemade chocolate yoghurt, you could add carob powder to live yoghurt. Instead of spaghetti hoops, you could cook up a pot of whole-wheat spaghetti and serve it with your own fresh tomato sauce. In place of garishly coloured fizzy drinks, give them orange juice mixed with sparkling water. But make the changes gradually. Be patient, persistent and as sneaky as you have to be. For instance, if your kids have always balked at eating vegetables, you can add peas and sautéed, pureed courgettes to their pasta sauce, or make vegetable soups that you put through the blender. (For detailed tips on making healthy changes in the kitchen, see Chapter 24.)

As ever, your own attitude to food is vitally important. If you're not keen on eating your greens, it's no surprise when your children follow suit! Notice your tone of voice when you offer different foods. You'll probably find that you present foods you yourself really like in an excited way. If carrots and broccoli don't sing to you, *you* need to get excited about vegetables too – and that might mean learning new ways to prepare them. *The Holford Low-GL Diet Cookbook*, co-authored by Patrick with Fiona McDonald Joyce, is a great way to start.

Ultimately, you'll need to eat well if you want your children to eat well. So the quest to optimally nourish your child will by necessity draw you in to this way of eating, too – which can hardly be a bad thing!

No bribes, rewards or punishments

Taking the emotion out of mealtimes can also help if you have a fussy eater. The majority of food fads are emotionally driven – often vehicles for your child to get attention or assert their independence. So the fewer emotions you display at the breakfast or dinner table, the better. For example, try not to praise your child lavishly for emptying their plate, and don't appear too hurt when your lovingly prepared vegetable casserole goes uneaten. Also, don't bribe or reward children with sweet foods, punish them for not eating, or force them to eat.

From the very start, eating should be a matter of satisfying appetite, not something you do for mummy (or even starving people). Nor does it need to be a tidy activity. So let your child's appetite, not your desire to feed them, be the governing factor at mealtimes. If they want more food one day, give it to them – they could be preparing for a growth spurt. Equally, if their hunger wanes the next day, don't force-feed them. They may be unwell or just tired.

Eating should also be an independent activity. As soon as your child can use spoon or hands – whichever is easier and (for their enjoyment) messier – encourage them to do so. So don't be too tough too soon on your child's manners. Let them learn to enjoy food first, and eat it tidily later.

Manage their choices

If your child is very young, it will be a few years before they can knowledgeably make a choice between, say, risotto or pasta. But while a toddler will not understand if you say 'What do you want for lunch today?', they may respond if you hold up an apple and a pear and say, 'Do you want an apple or a pear?' And with older children, it's better to give them a choice of two or three foods rather than asking the open question, 'What would you like to eat?'

Research by the British Food Council shows that children are more willing to eat the food they themselves have chosen. So while you need to keep this simple to avoid overwhelming your child or even encouraging fussiness, you can involve them more as they grow. For example, ask them to pick out some fruit and vegetables in the supermarket, or get them involved in preparing meals. Cooking for optimum nutrition is not only fun; it will also set them up for a lifetime of healthy eating, and give them a real alternative to the ubiquitous junk food that so many teenagers in the West succumb to.

Keep snacks simple

Snacks are important for keeping blood sugar even and energy stores topped up, but having too many may prevent your child from eating proper meals. If it looks as if this is happening, don't give interesting foods as snacks. If your child is really hungry between meals he or she will happily eat a carrot stick or an apple – so keep plenty of these in the fridge, and supply a sealed plastic box with crudités or a bit of fruit for schooldays too.

Note that drinking lots of milk can also dampen appetite, as it's a food and quite filling. If you notice your child is guzzling milk between meals, remind them that there's water or diluted fruit juice to drink, too.

Be careful, too, of rewarding or comforting your child with frequent snacks – this can lay down emotional patterns that may later encourage them to comfort eat when faced with a difficult situation which, in the long term, can lead to obesity. Three meals and two snacks a day, with raw vegetables and fresh fruit freely available, should keep them going.

Eating out

While you can provide your child with healthy food at home, keeping this up can be difficult when they visit friends or go to parties, or when your family eats out or goes on holiday. But as long as their basic diet is the best it can be, the occasional packet of crisps or bowl of chocolate ice cream is fine. And if you explain that there's one way of eating at home and another way elsewhere, you can help your child associate these 'treats' with special occasions and not pester you for them all the time. However, it's wise not to make this a big issue, or your child will begin to see certain foods as 'forbidden' – which will just enhance their appeal.

When you eat out in restaurants, you don't have to order food from a children's menu if all that it offers is fried and processed choices (nuggets and chips, for instance). Order an adult starter or share a main dish with your child, or ask to substitute the chips for a steamed vegetable or a salad. Also ask for diluted juices instead of fizzy drinks.

Combating food fussiness is not as difficult as it might seem.

- **Introduce a variety of foods as early as possible and set a good example.**

- **Remember, it's as much about psychology as nutrition. Be firm and consistent.**

CHAPTER 23

Guerrilla Tactics in the Supermarket

You'll have to face it sooner or later: what you want for your child and what the food manufacturers and marketers want are two different things. So you need to develop some guerrilla tactics in the supermarket, reading the labels carefully – and reading between the lines. The hopeful news is that, these days, there really is plenty of choice even in mainstream supermarkets. Add in what health food stores have to offer, and it just isn't that difficult to fill cupboard and fridge with wonderfully nutritious and delicious foods.

Here are the twelve golden shopping rules.

Avoid foods that contain hydrogenated fats

Check the label for the words 'hydrogenated' and 'vegetable oil'. If it contains vegetable oil and has a long shelf-life, the oil in the product has been hydrogenated – that is, processed so it hardens. As we discussed in Chapter 3, hydrogenated fats interfere with the brain's use of essential fats, and ultimately, with the smooth working of the brain.

Avoid foods that contain sugar

Check labels for sugar. This includes sucrose, glucose, dextrose, maltose and any other '-ose'. Sugars that won't play havoc with your child's blood glucose include xylitol, fructose and blue agave syrup, which is used in drinks. But only go for products where even these sugars are a long way down the ingredients list.

Avoid processed juice and fruit juice drinks

As discussed in Chapter 1, processed fruit juices and fruit juice drinks are no better than sugary water. With these products, don't be fooled by the manufacturers' assertions that the drink has been fortified with vitamins and minerals. All this means is that the original and natural nutrients have been destroyed through processing. The only acceptable juices are freshly made ones, or the kind that's kept in the chill cabinet and has a very short shelf life – just a few days, maximum. Apple juice is the best choice since apples contain mainly fructose.

Buy small blocks of cheese and small cartons of milk

Consuming a lot of dairy products can potentially trigger a sensitivity to these foods – milk is one of the top allergens, after all. Most cheese also has a lot of saturated fat. If you and your children are eating dairy products, don't buy family-sized blocks of cheese and 5-litre containers of milk – unless you are a family of 20! Buying smaller packages will keep your consumption down to a moderate level. Buy stronger-flavoured cheese such as Parmesan or mature Cheddar so that they can be used as a garnish rather than be eaten by the slab.

Choose free-range, organic and omega-3 rich eggs

Eggs are a superb brain food, but they're only as healthy as the chicken who laid them. If you can, buy omega-3 enriched eggs, preferably organic or at least free range.

Avoid foods that contain additives, preservatives and other chemicals

Check the list of nasties in Chapter 8, on page 87, and avoid these rigorously. There's also a list of the small number of healthy E numbers, which are actually vitamins, on page 87. As a good rule of thumb, a shorter ingredients list is likely to indicate a healthier food. For example, bread may have as few as three ingredients or as many as 30. Most importantly, if you read a long ingredients list and don't recognise many of these substances as 'food' – that is, something that grew on a tree or in the ground, for example – or you feel you could better recognise and pronounce them if you had a chemistry degree, this should sound the alarm bells that this product is not a good thing to give your child.

Make a list and stick to it

This is especially important if your child is going to the supermarket with you. You could write the list together. Use generic terms such as 'fruit and veg' so you're not limiting yourself and can pick what looks good. Don't put anything in the trolley that's not on the list, unless of course it's something you genuinely forgot you needed (and that clearly doesn't include chocolate biscuits!) If you are strict about this your child will accept it. Never cave in to your child's demands and don't be frightened of a tantrum. Caving in teaches them that a tantrum gets them exactly what they want. Avoid the biscuits and sweets aisle altogether. Remember, if they watch children's TV, every ad break is showcasing some refined, sugar-laden food that comes with small plastic gifts. Stay away from them!

Eat before you go shopping

And if your child is coming with you, give them a snack too. An apple and a few Brazil nuts in the car on the way to the supermarket will keep their blood sugar levels even. This deflects their cravings for sugary foods, and also prevents the irritability that goes along with it. Take a drink of water into the supermarket, too.

Buy organic when you can

Sometimes there is very little price difference between organic and non-organic foods, which is a boon. But be careful about organic processed foods. The ingredients are probably better quality, and it's likely to be E number-free, but organic pizza and chips are still pizza and chips, and organic cake can still be laden with sugar. And as we've seen, refined carbohydrates add nothing to a healthy diet.

Choose whole foods over refined and processed

This means brown rice, wholemeal pasta, and wholegrain bread instead of white. Choose whole vegetables, not ready-prepared vegetables – these will have been haemorrhaging nutrients since they were sliced. It's better, and much cheaper, to buy a whole lettuce or cabbage than to buy prepared salads or salad greens that are likely to have been 'treated' and will start to go off within minutes of opening the bag.

Variety is the spice of life

Be adventurous and try new things, especially fresh produce and pulses. Have you ever eaten quinoa or pearl barley, or had grated beetroot raw in a salad? Variety is key to good nutrition and makes mealtimes a lot more pleasurable, too.

Watch out for '95% fat free'

As we discussed in Chapter 3, fat phobia is misguided. It's the *type* of fat that counts. Most products that claim to be low-fat have had sugar added to make them palatable, so they're not any better (and probably worse) than the original. Watch out for reduced-fat items where the original item is actually a naturally high-fat food. An example is low-fat butter. Butter is supposed to be virtually 100 per cent fat, so check the ingredients list to see what's been added instead.

CHAPTER 24

Top Tips in the Kitchen

If your child has developed a taste for less-than-healthy foods, you'll need to change their diet. Does even the idea fill you with foreboding? Don't worry: although it can be tough weaning them off double-cheese pizzas and 'chips with everything', this chapter shows it can be done gradually and relatively painlessly, all round.

For example, if your child refuses to eat vegetables but will eat tomato sauce, begin by adding small amounts of pureed vegetables to the sauce, and increase teaspoon by teaspoon over the days and weeks. This way, they simply won't notice the changing taste and appearance – but within three months will actually be eating a highly nutritious, vitamin-rich sauce with their pasta. Their tastebuds will have become used to the vegetables. After this, it's simply a case of blending the vegetables less and less thoroughly so they get chunkier over time. When you finally present a plate of vegetables to your child, their tastebuds will register them as a familiar food and they are more likely to actually enjoy eating them.

For children who will only eat fish fingers and chicken nuggets, begin by making your own. Try to make them look similar to the commercial varieties. With these, too, you can begin to add pureed steamed vegetables, pureed boiled lentils or pureed tins of beans to the fish or chicken mixture. Add tiny amounts at the start, then increase gradually. Eventually, your child will be eating lentil and vegetable fingers and burgers that are rich in nutrients and fibre instead of packaged food that may be of dubious quality and devoid of nutrients.

This is not to say that retraining tastebuds isn't difficult. One of the biggest problems with getting kids who eat a lot of junk food to switch to healthy wholefoods is the powerful artificial flavours and additives lurking in so many highly processed products. Wholefoods can seem very bland by comparison at the start, but perseverance, the gradual introduction of healthy ingredients as outlined above, and a clever use of herbs, spices, nutritious oils, lemon juice and the like can work wonders.

Here are a few useful guidelines:

- If your child insists that he or she really doesn't like peas, for example, tell them they only have to eat three peas. (Although if they say this about every vegetable you serve, it's time to move on to the gradual-introduction method outlined above.)

- Steaming vegetables is the best cooking method. Steamed vegetables taste better and retain more nutrients than boiled, and are healthier than fried. Adding a drizzle of olive oil, a knob of butter or a squeeze of lemon juice really boosts their flavour too. Or you can steam-fry them – sauté the chosen veg briefly, add a tablespoon of soy sauce, water or stock, and clamp the lid on till they're steamed.

- Get your children involved in food preparation as early in life as possible. From a very young age, they can sprinkle seeds on a salad, for example.

- Many children will happily eat raw vegetables rather than cooked, so capitalise on this by providing raw veg as pre-dinner snacks.

So what, specifically, should you be feeding your child for optimum brain health?

The best breakfasts

To get your child off to the best start in the day, you can ring the changes on three basic options – cereal, a cooked breakfast or toast.

Cereal

The best is porridge (cooked oats) or muesli (raw oats) with plenty of nuts and seeds and fresh fruit (grated apple or diced ripe pear or plums are excellent). Serve with dairy, soya, rice or quinoa milk. Watch out for boxed mueslis that are loaded with hidden sugar or a lot of dried fruit. Muesli shouldn't taste sweet. The sweetness comes from the fresh fruit you add.

Cooked breakfast

Poached or scrambled eggs, or kippers (smoked herring), are excellent, either served with wholegrain bread. Choose bread that most closely resembles a housebrick and has visible whole grains. Heavy and hard breads contain less yeast, which is better for blood sugar balance and also for digestive health. Some 'brown' breads are only brown because of added colouring!

Toast

Again, heavy, grainy breads are the best choice. Rather than loads of sugary jams or marmalade, top with protein. You don't want to send your child out the door on a sugar high, only for them to slump an hour later at school. So give them hummus, avocado or nut butters (almond, hazelnut and cashew make a nice change from peanut, and pumpkin seed butter is superb, but whatever kind you go for, ensure it doesn't contain sweetener). The only jams your child should have should be sugar-free and loaded with fruit, such as blueberries.

Unless your child is allergic to dairy, butter is a better bet than margarine or any of the other alternative spreads. If your child is allergic to dairy, then pumpkin seed butter or tahini (made from sesame seeds and their oil) are the best non-dairy spreads.

Lunch and dinner - the template

With breakfast sorted, how should you approach lunch and dinner? If you think of a plate and how to fill it, both these meals should be about a quarter protein, a quarter starchy carbohydrates and the remaining half vegetables and/or salad. Protein-rich foods are fish, eggs, meat, pulses (lentils and beans), quinoa, and nuts and seeds; starchy carbohydrates include bread, pasta, rice, potato, sweet potato and corn; and vegetables are all other vegetables, whether eaten cooked or raw. These proportions should apply whether the foods sit separately on the plate or are combined into a soup, stew or main-meal tossed salad.

If the protein doesn't include some essential fats from nuts, seeds or oily fish, simply add some by drizzling some good-quality cold-pressed seed oil on the vegetables or salad, or sprinkling on a garnish of ground seeds. (See the next chapter for ideas on school lunches and how to fill their lunch boxes with zingy, supernutritious foods.)

Two-day menu

Breakfast	*Breakfast*
Porridge with chopped plum and seeds	Wholegrain toast with almond butter
Snack	*Snack*
An apple and a handful of raw cashews	A pear and some pumpkin seeds
Lunch	*Lunch*
Spaghetti bolognese with puréed vegetables hidden in the sauce	Pasta shapes with a chicken and tomato sauce Carrot and celery sticks
Snack	*Snack*
Sugar snap peas and cherry tomatoes	Oat biscuits and a kiwi
Dinner	*Dinner*
Fish, mashed potatoes, broccoli and French beans	Stew with chickpeas and a variety of vegetables
Drinks throughout the day Diluted fresh fruit juice or water	*Drinks throughout the day* Diluted fresh fruit juice or water

---

Finger on the pulse

Lentils and beans may not be a food you grew up with, but they certainly deserve a prominent place in your family's diet. A great source of protein, they also add fibre and important nutrients, help hormonal balance, and are economical to boot – helping offset some of the costs you may incur through buying organic, for instance. As cultures from India to Mexico know, they're also delicious and wonderfully versatile to cook with. You can use them to enliven a massive range of soups, stew, salads, veggie burgers, veggie dips and sandwich fillings – the list is endless.

Lentils are cooked from dry in a mere 15 to 30 minutes, depending on the variety. Beans and chickpeas can be bought in tins from any supermarket (look for those packed in water, without sugar or salt), and just need rinsing before use. Or if you're really keen you can buy them dried, soak overnight and boil for the time indicated on the packet. Note that pulses need to be chewed thoroughly, as otherwise they can cause gas.

All pulses (excluding the 'split' kind) can also be sprouted, making a tasty and amazingly nutritious addition to salads and sandwiches. As the sprouting process only takes three or four days, your child might enjoy growing their own food and experiencing the excitement of watching its progress, day by day.

Choosing fats and oils for cooking

If you must fry, far and away the best cooking oil is coconut. Despite its lardy appearance at fridge or room temperature, coconut oil is a very healthy choice because it cannot be harmed by heating. The medium-chain triglycerides or MCTs it contains are also much easier for the body to burn for energy, so it's less likely to be stored as fat. And don't worry – it has no flavour of its own. The next best option is butter, unless you're dairy-free, followed by olive oil (a monounsaturated fat), which is slightly damaged by frying.

Whichever you use, never fry at high heat. Steam-frying is much better, as we've seen. With onions and garlic, for instance, sauté them in your chosen oil just enough to generate heat and then soften slightly; then add in the other ingredients and a dash of water, stock or soy sauce. Clamp the lid on and steam gently for a few minutes. With this method, the temperature – and the nutrient loss – are much lower.

And if you want to give soups, stews and curries a rich, creamy touch, you don't have to go for cream; coconut milk or a dab of hummus or tahini are healthy dairy-free options.

There are lots of quick, easy and delicious recipes using all these principles in *The Optimum Nutrition Cookbook* and *The Holford Low-GL Diet Cookbook.*

CHAPTER 25

Making Healthy Meals at School Cool

 Once your child starts attending nursery or school, or spends time with a child carer, your control of their diet begins to slip away. Essentially, your child will either be eating the packed lunch that you supply, or a school meal. Things are improving there, spurred on by Jamie Oliver's graphic demonstration that school meals can be good without costing the earth, and the government's recent commitment to up spending on them. But there's no way round it: you still need to be sure of what your kids are eating when you're not around.

At nursery or school

It's particularly important to check out nurseries, because young children aren't really up to making a lot of choices about food. Before you commit to one, find out what they will be feeding your child. If it doesn't impress, look elsewhere or see if they're focusing on healthy food, or in the process of doing something about it. If parents demand better food for their children, it will be provided – there's nothing as effective for change as voting with your feet.

At school, however, what a child eats is likely to be completely up to them. If your child already has an appetite for healthy food, then they are more likely to make healthy choices. If not, then it is doubly important that the choices on offer are good.

We find that when working with children who choose their own lunch at school, it's important that they have a good incentive to eat healthily. Prevention of heart disease in later life is unlikely to impress a 10-year-old much: that's just too far into the future for them to be able to take on board. But if you tell them it will help them be a better football player, have more friends, do better in class, stop getting into trouble and have clear skin, that's much more motivating.

Optimum nutrition improves health and well-being on myriad levels, but you need to focus on what's important to your child. After all, being better at maths is not much of an incentive to an artistic child who has no interest in maths.

Breakfast clubs

As we saw in Chapter 12, these clubs are theoretically a great idea, and they're springing up all over the country. But if you need to use this service, you'll need to take a hard look at what's on the menu before you allow your child to go for it. If 'breakfast' is sugary cereal, white toast, jam and juice drinks, you're effectively putting your child on a blood sugar roller-coaster. So you have two choices: exert your influence as a concerned parent to ensure that better breakfast options (outlined in Chapter 24) are available, or give your child break-fast at home.

The optimum lunch box and snacks

When you're putting your child's lunch box and snacks together for the day, follow the lunch and dinner templates on page 241, as these supply the best range of nutrients and best blood sugar balance. A couple of peanut butter sandwiches on wholegrain bread with a simple salad fits the bill.

A salad box is a great alternative to sandwiches in summer, but make sure it contains enough protein and quality carbohydrates. An active child cannot get through the day on lettuce leaves. Try tuna and pasta salad with carrot and celery sticks and some sugarsnap peas. Or falafel, or lentil burgers, with brown basmati rice salad and cherry tomatoes, baby corn and sprouts. In winter, a flask of thick, hearty soup is wonderful – just be sure to follow the proportions in the lunch and dinner templates when you're making it.

Great snacks include fresh fruit, nuts and seeds, oatcakes, crudités or savoury muffins (made with chickpea flour, for example). As for drinks, it seems most children will drink water quite happily if it's in a 'sports' bottle, so pop in one of those full of water or diluted fruit juice each day.

So, to recap – what might go into that packed lunch? Try a hummus and salad sandwich on wholegrain rye bread, a peanut butter sandwich on wholegrain oat bread, some carrot sticks, an apple, some brazil nuts, a couple of oatcakes and a bottle of water.

On the way to and from school

Once your child has their own money and is walking to school on their own, you can't stop them from buying sweets at the shop on the way to or from school. However, if their schoolbag is full of healthy snacks and their pockets are not full of money, you will have less to worry about. Also, if they've had a good breakfast at home, they'll be less inclined to buy food on the way to school. And if they're used to nutritious, wholesome food and have balanced blood sugar, they will be less inclined to gorge on the really unhealthy stuff.

So keep a check on it but try not to make it a big deal. On

the whole, the food your child eats will be what you provide for them at home, and that is what's most important.

Help your school feed your child properly

If you'd like to get moving on helping your child's school improve the food they serve, there are a number of websites that you can share with the school. First is a government website, www.foodinschools.org, that advises schools on how to work on this area. The Soil Association have an excellent downloadable guide for schools called Food for Life (www.soilassociation.org/foodforlife). Give this to the head of your child's school. Jamie Oliver's website www.feedmebetter.com provides more helpful information for transforming school meals, focusing on using fresh ingredients. And there is a charity working to link education and lifelong learning with health – www.continyou.org.uk. They provide some excellent practical advice for setting up breakfast clubs.

All of these are resources that have made a huge impact already on the food children eat in school. We don't think they go far enough, however – so we have launched Food for the Brain – an educational charity promoting optimum nutrition for schoolchildren's minds. The Food for the Brain schools campaign (www.foodforthebrain.org), explained in Chapter 27, also gives schools and parents advice on how to boost the quality of school meals. Make sure your child's school signs up.

CHAPTER 26

Supplements for Superkids

 We've demonstrated throughout this book that a varied and nutritious diet is the keystone of good mental and emotional health. But sometimes even the best diets fail to provide appropriate levels of all the nutrients we need, and some children need more of certain nutrients than others. Also, as we've seen, children can be very picky eaters. Add to that the logistical challenge of providing a day's meals perfectly balanced in every nutrient, and what you're looking at is supplements.

Supplementation is the most reliable way to ensure your child gets appropriate levels of all the vitamins and minerals they need to be optimally nourished. This is even more important if your child is having a hard time of it mentally or emotionally. Remember that there's a range of vitamins and minerals essential for good health, and a small deficiency in any one nutrient could have a serious impact on your growing child.

When to start supplementing

As soon as you start weaning your child, it's worth supplementing. As long as you're breastfeeding, it's you that needs to take the supplemental nutrients, which then get passed on to them naturally.

The chart below shows the ideal daily amounts of vitamins, minerals and essential fats to supplement from weaning to age 13, assuming you are feeding them a reasonably health diet. Once a child is 14, adult amount of nutrients apply. You can find these in Chapter 45 of the *New Optimum Nutrition Bible* or at www.patrickholford.com/content.asp?id_ Content=1206.

The ideal daily supplement programme

Age Nutrient	Less than 1	1–2	3–4	5–6	7–8	9–11	12–13
Essential vitamins							
A (retinol)	500mcg	650	800	1,000	1,500	2,000	2,500
D	1mcg	1.4	1.75	2.25	2.5	2.75	3.0
E	13mg	16	20	23	30	40	50
C	100mg	150	300	400	500	600	700
B1 (thiamine)	5mg	6	8	12	16	20	24
B2 (riboflavin)	5 mg	6	8	12	16	20	24
B3 (niacin)	7mg	12	16	18	20	22	24
B5 (pantothenic acid)	10mg	15	20	25	30	35	40
B6 (pyridoxine)	5mg	7	10	12	16	20	25
B12	5mcg	6.5	8	9	10	10	10
Folic acid	100mcg	120	140	160	180	200	220
Biotin	30mcg	45	60	70	80	90	100
Essential minerals							
Calcium	150mg	165	180	190	200	210	220
Magnesium	50mg	65	80	90	100	110	120
Iron	4mg	5.5	7	8	9	10	10
Zinc	4mg	5.5	7	8	9	10	10
Manganese	300mcg	350	400	500	700	1,000	1,000
Iodine	40mcg	50	60	70	80	90	100
Chromium	15mcg	19	23	25	27	30	30
Selenium	10mcg	18	20	24	26	28	30
Copper	400mcg	550	700	800	900	1,000	1,000

Age	Less than 1	1–2	3–4	5–6	7–8	9–11	12–13
Nutrient							
Essential fats							
GLA	50	75	95	110	135	135	135
EPA	100	175	250	300	350	350	350
DHA	100	140	175	200	225	225	225

Other brain nutrients (optional)	
Phosphatidyl choline	250 to 400mg
Phosphatidyl serine	20 to 45mg
DMAE	200 to 300mg
Glutamine	250 to 1000mg
Arginine pyroglutamate	300 to 450mg
Trimethyl glycine (TMG)	250mg–1000mg

Choosing the right supplements

With supplements for your child, you're looking at three broad areas: multis, essential fats and, if needed, extra brain nutrients.

Finding a good multi

Many companies formulate single multivitamin and mineral supplements that incorporate all the necessary nutrients especially for children (see Resources, page 280). The chart above will give you guidelines on the levels of nutrients to look for. You can choose chewable (or crushable in the early stages) or liquid or soluble formulas, depending on your (or your child's) preferences.

You should ideally give your child his or her supplement with breakfast, but certainly not last thing at night, as the B vitamins can have a mild stimulatory effect. (For some children, glutamine can also be stimulating.) Children also tend to be more susceptible to vitamin toxicity than adults, and while the doses listed are well within any potentially toxic limits for even the most sensitive child, don't be tempted to give much more than these recommended levels unless under the direction and supervision of a nutritional therapist.

Unless you are trying to correct a specific problem and giving glutamine powder, or probiotics, in most cases you'll choose a chewable multivitamin and mineral, usually giving one for every two years of life. So, by the time your child is eight they'll be taking four a day. (Of course, this depends on the amount of vitamins and minerals in the supplements, so check levels against our guidelines on page 250.) These are best spread out, perhaps two with breakfast and two with lunch. Few chewable multis contain enough vitamin C, zinc, calcium or magnesium. This is because vitamin C tastes tart, zinc tastes metallic, and calcium and magnesium make chewables crunchy – and less chewable!

There are a number of ways to get round this problem. Assuming you are giving your child ground seeds every day, as we recommend, these will guarantee a reasonable amount of zinc, calcium and magnesium. You can get powdered calcium/magnesium to add to drinks, or a chewable vitamin C that uses calcium/magnesium ascorbate, thus killing three birds with one stone. If your child doesn't sleep well, and a little extra magnesium would help, this is a good option. The best way to give your child a little extra vitamin C is to make sure they eat at least five servings of fruit and vegetables a day. The best foods for vitamin C are peppers, broccoli, berries and citrus fruit.

If need be, you can always crush any supplement and add it to water or diluted fruit juice.

Essential fats to boost IQ

As long as your child is eating oily fish three times a week and a daily portion of seeds, they should be getting a good background level of essential fats to help their brains develop and boost IQ. However, if they don't eat fish or don't have seeds every day, we recommend you supplement their diet with an essential fat formula. Look for one that contains both GLA (omega-6) and DHA and EPA, which are the most important omega-3 fats for development (see Resources, page 280). The most important essential fat is omega-3 and there are many different forms of supplements supplying this essential fat on the market, ranging from pastes to drinks to tiny capsules. You can always pierce a capsule and add it to juice or food.

The chart above gives you the rough quantities to aim for in a supplement, assuming they are receiving the same again from seeds and the occasional serving of oily fish.

Extra brain nutrients

In addition to the essential vitamins, minerals and essential fats, we've also extolled the virtues of phospholipids (phosphatidyl choline, serine and DMAE), as well as glutamine and its cousin pyroglutamate. These can be supplemented as well (see Resources, page 280), but they usually come in tablets that might be hard for a younger child to swallow. For phosphatidyl choline (PC) you can add some lecithin granules to cereal, generally giving a dessertspoon of regular lecithin or a teaspoonful of hi-PC lecithin. Glutamine also comes in powder that easily dissolves in water or diluted juice.

To ensure your child is getting enough brain-boosting nutrients, there are several easy steps you can take.

- Give your child a good multivitamin and multimineral formula based on the nutrient levels given in this chapter.

- Give your child an omega-3 fish oil supplement every day.

- If your child is struggling, look for a specific 'brain food' formula with additional brain nutrients listed above.

CHAPTER 27

Join the Food for the Brain Campaign

It's in childhood that we build the rest of our lives – yet it sometimes seems as if there are too many pitfalls on this journey. You have no doubt despaired at the quality of school meals, the junk designed to fill kids' lunch boxes, and the vast, ever-expanding variety of sugary drinks and snacks crowding the supermarket shelves. You've probably wondered why something as important as optimum nutrition isn't taught in schools so all children can learn how what they eat affects their health and their mind. You've no doubt wondered why legislators aren't doing more to act on the obvious link between poor diet and increasing behavioural problems and crime.

To put this into context, last year an estimated £342 million was spent on school behaviour improvement programmes for children with behavioural problems, but nutrition failed to figure at all in this programme. No government departments have yet made any commitment, or committed any funds, to research or promote optimum nutrition for your child's mind.

You might wish there was a way to make this change, or a way you could make a difference. There is. It's called the

Food for the Brain Campaign, which we mentioned in Chapter 25.

Together with many of the world's leading experts in nutrition and behaviour, scientists whose work we have quoted in this book, and pioneering charities, we've initiated a campaign whose mission is

> to promote the awareness of the link between nutrition and mental health. To educate children, parents, teachers, schools, the public and professionals about optimum nutrition for mental health. To give schools, members of the public and health professionals access to educational material and services promoting mental health through optimum nutrition.

The Food for the Brain Campaign is something that you can both benefit from and participate in.

- Visit the website www.foodforthebrain.org and sign up for the free e-news to keep informed of all the latest information about how to keep yourself and your child in the best of health.

- Find out how you can encourage your child's school to join the Food for the Brain Campaign instigating a policy of no sugary drinks and snacks and better school meals and lunch boxes.

- Invite a nutritional therapist to present a lecture at your child's school – one for the parents and teachers, one for the children themselves.

- Support our campaign to advance the research in this vital area – and get it put into practice by volunteering, or taking part in fund-raising activities, or becoming a supporting member of the Food for the Brain Campaign, for as little as £10 a year.

- Tell your friends to visit the website www.foodforthe-brain.org and read this book.

Above all, remember – you are not alone. More and more parents like you, teachers, schools, doctors, politicians and children are waking up to the fact that what you eat not only has a profound effect on your physical health but also how you think and feel. By joining the Food for the Brain Campaign, you're helping create a better world in the future for our children, and our children's children.

Wishing you health and happiness,

Patrick Holford and Deborah Colson

REFERENCES

1   D. Benton and G. Roberts, 'Effect of vitamin and mineral supple-
    mentation on intelligence of school children', *Lancet*, Vol 1(8578),
    1988, pp. 140–3

2   B. Gesch, 'Influence of supplementary vitamins, minerals and essential
    fats on the antisocial behaviour of young adult prisoners', *British
    Journal of Psychiatry*, Vol 181, 2002, pp. 22–8

3   A. J. Richardson and P. Montgomery, 'The Oxford-Durham study: A
    randomized controlled trial of dietary supplementation with fatty
    acids in children with developmental coordination disorder',
    Pediatrics, Vol 115, 2005, pp. 1360–6

4   A. Borjel *et al.*, *Homocysteine Metabolism*, 5th International Conference
    Abstract, Italy, June 2005.

5   C. M. Carter *et al.*, 'Effects of a few food diet in attention deficit
    disorder', *Archives of Disease in Childhood*, Vol 69, 1993, pp. 564–8

6   Survey by Dr Bernard Rimland. *www.autismwebsite.com/
    ari/treatment/form34q.htm*

7   World Health Organization, *The World Health Report 2001 – Mental
    Health: New Understanding, New Hope*, WHO, 2001. Available at
    www.who.int/whr/2001/

8   A. K. Borjel *et al.*, 'Plasma homocysteine levels, MTHFR polymor-
    phisms 677C>T, 1298A>C, 1793G>A, and school achievement in a
    population sample of Swedish children', paper presented at
    Homocysteine Metabolism, 5th International Conference, Milano
    (Italy), June 26–30, 2005

9   J. Penland, Experimental Biology conference, San Diego, April 4, 2005
    (pending publication)

10 A. G. Schauss, 'Nutrition and behavior', *Journal of Applied Nutrition*, vol
    35(1), pp. 30–5 (1983)

11 D. Benton *et al.*, 'The impact of the supply of glucose to the brain on
    mood and memory', *Nutrition Reviews*, Vol 59(1 Pt 2), 2001, pp. S20–1

12 D. Benton *et al.*, 'Mild hypoglycaemia and questionnaire measures of
    aggression', *Biological Psychology*, Vol 14(1–2), 1982, pp. 129–35

13   A. Roy *et al.*, 'Monoamines, glucose metabolism, aggression toward self and others', *International Journal of Neuroscience*, Vol 41(3–4), 1988, pp. 261–4

14   A. G. Schauss, *Diet, Crime and Delinquency*, Parker House, 1980

15   M. Virkkunen, 'Reactive hypoglycaemic tendency among arsonists', *Acta Psychiatrica Scandinavica*, Vol 69(5), 1984, pp. 445–52

16   M. Virkkunen and S. Narvanen, 'Tryptophan and serotonin levels during the glucose tolerance test among habitually violent and impulsive offenders', *Neuropsychobiology*, Vol 17(1–2), 1987, pp. 19–23

17   J. Yaryura-Tobias and F. Neziroglu, 'Violent behaviour, Brain dysrythmia and glucose dysfunction: A new syndrome', *Journal of Orthomolecular Psychiatry*, Vol 4, 1975, pp. 182–5

18   M. Bruce and M. Lader, 'Caffeine abstention and the management of anxiety disorders', *Psychological Medicine*, Vol 19, 1989, pp. 211–14

19   W. Wendel and W. Beebe, 'Glycolytic activity in schizophrenia', in D. Hawkins and L. Pauling (eds), *Orthomolecular Psychiatry*, 1973

20   R. Prinz and D. Riddle, 'Associations between nutrition and behaviour in 5 year old children', *Nutrition Reviews*, Vol 43, suppl., 1986

21   L. Christensen, 'Psychological distress and diet – effects of sucrose and caffeine', *Journal of Applied Nutrition*, Vol 40(1), 1988, pp. 44–50

22   D. Fullerton *et al.*, 'Sugar, opionoids and binge eating', *Brain Research Bulletin*, Vol 14(6), 1985, pp. 273–80

23   L. Christensen, 'Psychological distress and diet: Effects of sucrose and caffeine', *Journal of Applied Nutrition*, Vol 40, 1988, pp. 44–50

24   M. Colgan and L. Colgan, 'Do nutrient supplements and dietary changes affect learning and emotional reactions of children with learning difficulties? A controlled series of 16 cases', *Nutritional Health*, Vol 3, 1984, pp. 69–77

25   J. Goldman *et al.*, 'Behavioural effects of sucrose on preschool children', *J Abnormal Child Psychology*, Vol 14(4), 1986, pp. 565–77

26   M. Lester *et al.*, 'Refined carbohydrate intake, hair cadmium levels and cognitive functioning in children', *Nutrition and Behaviour*, Vol 1, 1982, pp. 3–13

27   S. Schoenthaler *et al.*, 'The impact of low food additive and sucrose diet on academic performance in 803 New York City public schools', *International Journal of Biosocial Research*, Vol 8(2), 1986, pp. 185–95

28   R. J. Prinz *et al.*, 'Dietary correlates of hyperactive behaviour in children', *Journal of Consulting and Clinical Psychology*, Vol 48, 1980, pp. 760–9

29   S. J. Schoenthaler *et al.*, 'The effect of randomised vitamin-mineral supplementation on violent and non-violent antisocial behaviour among

incarcerated juveniles', *Journal of Nutritional and Environmental Medicine*, Vol 7, 1997, pp 343–52

30 L. Langseth and J. Dowd, 'Glucose tolerance and hyperkinesis', *Food and Cosmetics Toxicology*, Vol 16, 1978, p. 129

31 R. G. Walton *et al.*, 'Adverse reactions to aspartame: Double blind challenge in patients from a vulnerable population', *Biological Psychiatry*, Vol 34(1–2), 1993, pp.13–17

32 Wesnes, K.A. *et al.*, 'Breakfast reduces declines in attention and memory over the morning in schoolchildren', *Appetite*, Vol 41, 2003, pp. 329–31

33 K. Gilliland and D. Andress, 'Ad lib caffeine consumption, symptoms of caffeinism, and academic performance', *American Journal of Psychiatry*, Vol 138(4), 1981, pp. 512–14

34 N. J. Richardson *et al.*, 'Mood and performance effects of caffeine in relation to acute and chronic caffeine deprivation', *Pharmacology, Biochemistry and Behavior*, Vol 52(2), 1995, pp. 313–20

35 M. Makrides, 'Are long-chain polyunsaturated fatty acids essential nutrients in infancy?' *Lancet*, Vol 345, 1995, pp.1463–8

36 L. Stevens, 'Essential fat metabolism in boys with attention-deficit hyperactivity disorder', *American Journal of Clinical Nutrition*, Vol 62, 1995, pp.761–8

37 P. Willatts *et al.*, 'Effect of long-chain polyunsaturated fatty acids in infant formula on problem solving at 10 months of age', *Lancet*, Vol 352, 1998, pp. 688–91

38 J. B. Helland *et al.*, 'Maternal supplementation with very-long-chain n-3 fatty acids during pregnancy and lactation augments children's IQ at 4 years of age', *Pediatrics*, Vol 111, 2003, pp. 39–44

39 A. Richardson and B. Puri, 'A randomized double-blind, placebo-controlled study of the effects of supplementation with highly unsaturated fatty acids on ADHD-related symptoms in children with specific learning difficulties', *Progress in Neuro-Psychopharmacology and Biological Psychiatry*, Vol 26(2), 2002, pp 233–9

40 A. J. Richardson and P. Montgomery, 'The Oxford-Durham study: A randomized controlled trial of dietary supplementation with fatty acids in children with developmental coordination disorder', *Pediatrics*, Vol 115, 2005, pp. 1360–6

41 L. J. Stevens *et al.*, 'Essential fat metabolism in boys with attention-deficit hyperactivity disorder', *American Journal of Clinical Nutrition*, Vol 65, 1995, pp. 761–8

42 J. R. Burgess, *ADHD: observational and interventional studies*, NIH workshop on omega-3 EFAs in psychiatric disorders, National Institutes of Health, Bethesda, Maryland, US, 1988

43   A. J. Richardson *et al.*, *Treatment with highly unsaturated fatty acids can reduce ADHD symptoms in children with specific learning difficulties: A randomised controlled trial*, paper given at British Dyslexia Association International Conference, University of York, UK, April 2001

44   A. Richardson and B. Puri, 'A randomized double-blind, placebo-controlled study of the effects of supplementation with highly unsaturated fatty acids on ADHD-related symptoms in children with specific learning difficulties', *Progress in Neuro-Psychopharmacology and Biological Psychiatry*, Vol 26(2), 2002, pp. 233–9

45   S. E. Carlson *et al.*, 'Long-term feeding of formulas high in linolenic acid and marine oil to very low birth weight infants: Phospholipids fatty acids', *Pediatric Research*, Vol 30, 1991, pp. 404–12

46   A. J. Richardson and P. Montgomery, 'The Oxford-Durham study', *Pediatrics*, 2005

47   G. Pyapali *et al.*, 'Prenatal dietary choline supplementation', *Journal of Neurophysiology*, Vol 79(4), pp. 1790–6 and W. H. Meck *et al.*, *Neuroreport*, Vol 8, 1998, 1997, pp. 2831–5

48   S.Y. Chung *et al.*, 'Administration of phosphatidylcholine increases brain acetylcholine concentration and improves memory in mice with dementia', *Journal of Nutrition*, Vol 125(6), 1995, pp. 1484–9

49   R. J. Wurtman and S. H. Zeisel, 'Brain choline: Its sources and effects on the synthesis and release of acetylcholine', *Aging*, Vol 19, 1982, pp. 303–13

50   W. Poldinger *et al.*, 'A functional-dimensional approach to depression: Serotonin deficiency and target syndrome in a comparison of 5–hydroxytryptophan and fluvoxamine', *Psychopathology*, Vol 24(2), 1991, pp. 53–81

51   J. B. Deijen *et al.*, 'Tyrosine improves cognitive performance and reduces blood pressure in cadets', *Brain Research Bulletin*, Vol 48(2), 1999, pp. 203–9

52   I. S. Shiah and N.Yatham, 'GABA functions in mood disorders: An update and critical review', *Nature Life Sciences*, Vol 63(15) 1998, pp. 1289–1303

53   D. Benton and G. Roberts, 'Effect of vitamin and mineral supplementation on intelligence of school children', *Lancet*, 1998

54   A. Lucas *et al.*, 'Randomised trial of early diet in preterm babies and later intelligence quotient', *BMJ*, Vol 317, 1998, pp. 1481–7

55   A Borjel *et al.*, *Homocysteine Metabolism*, June 2005

56   D. Benton *et al.*, 'The impact of long-term vitamin supplementation on cognitive functioning', *Psychopharmacology* (Berl), Vol 117(3), 1995, pp. 298–305

57   D. Benton *et al.*, 'Thiamine supplementation, mood and cognitive functioning', *Psychopharmacol* (Berl), Vol 129(1), 1997, pp. 66–71

58 M. Louwman *et al.*, 'Signs of impaired cognitive function in adolescents with marginal cobalamin status', *American Journal of Clinical Nutrition*, Vol 72, 2000, pp. 762–9

59 J. Greenblatt *et al.*, 'Folic acid in neurodevelopment and child psychiatry', *Progress in Neuro-Psychopharmacology and Biological Psychiatry*, Vol 18(4), 1994, pp. 647–60

60 S. Johnson, 'Micronutrient accumulation and depletion in schizophrenia, epilepsy, autism and Parkinson's disease?', *Medical Hypotheses*, Vol 56(5), 2002, pp. 641–5

61 J. Penland, Experimental Biology conference, San Diego, April 4, 2005 (pending publication)

62 H. L. Needleman *et al.*, 'The long-term effects of exposure to low doses of lead in childhood: An 11–year follow-up report', *New England Journal of Medicine*, Vol 332, 1990, pp. 83–8

63 S. Davies, Editorial, *Journal of Nutritional Medicine*, Vol 2(3), 1991, pp. 227–47

64 N. I. Ward *et al.*, 'The influence of the chemical additive tartrazine on the zinc status of hyperactive children – a double-blind placebo controlled study', *Journal of Nutritional Medicine*, Vol 1, 1990, pp. 51–7

65 B. Bateman *et al.*, 'The effects of a double blind, placebo controlled, artificial food colourings and benzoate preservative challenge on hyperactivity in a general population sample of preschool children', *Archives of Disease in Childhood*, Vol 89, 2004, pp. 506–11

66 E. Young *et al.*, 'A population study of food intolerance', *Lancet*, Vol 343, 1994, pp. 1127–9

67 British Society for Allergy and Environmental Medicine, *Effective Allergy Practice*, 1984

68 T. Randolph, 'Allergy as a causative factor of fatigue, irritability and behaviour problems of children', *J Pediatr*, Vol 31, 1947, p. 560

69 A. Rowe, 'Allergic toxemia and fatigue', *Annals of Allergy*, Vol 17, 1959, p. 9

70 F. Speer, ed., 'Etiology: Foods', in *Allergy of the Nervous System*, Charles Thomas, 1970

71 M. Campbell, 'Neurologic manifestations of allergic disease', *Annals of Allergy*, Vol 31, 1973, p. 485

72 K. Hall, 'Allergy of the nervous system: A review', *Annals of Allergy*, Vol 36, 1976, pp. 49–64

73 V. Pippere, 'Some varieties of food intolerance in psychiatric patients', *Nutritional Health*, Vol 3(3), 1984, pp. 125–136

74 C. Pfeiffer and P. Holford, *Mental Illness and Schizophrenia: The nutrition connection*, Thorsons, 1989

75 T. Tuormaa, *An Alternative to Psychiatry*, The Book Guild, 1991

76 J. Egger *et al.*, 'Controlled trial of oligoantigenic treatment in the hyperkinetic syndrome', *Lancet*, 9 March 1985, pp. 540–5

77 J. Egger *et al.*, 'Is migraine a food allergy? A double-blind controlled trial of oligoantigenic diet treatment', *Lancet*, 15 October 1983, pp. 865–9

78 A. L. Kubala and M. M. Katz, 'Nutritional factors in psychological test behaviour', *J Genet Psychol*, Vol 96, 1960, pp. 343–52

79 R. F. Harrell *et al.*, 'Can nutritional supplements help mentally retarded children? An exploratory study', *Proceedings of the National Academy of Sciences* USA, Vol 78(1), 1981, pp. 574–8

80 D. Benton and G. Roberts, 'Effect of vitamin and mineral supplementation on intelligence of school children', *Lancet*, 1988

81 S. J. Schoenthaler *et al.*, 'Controlled trial of vitamin-mineral supplementation: Effects on intelligence and performance', *Personality and Individual Differences*, Vol 12(4), 1991, pp. 351–2

82 D. Benton, 'Micro-nutrient supplementation and the intelligence of children', *Neuroscience and Biobehavioral Reviews*, Vol 25(4), 2001, pp. 297–309

83 M. Nelson *et al.*, 'Nutrient intakes, vitamin-mineral supplementation and intelligence in British schoolchildren', *British Journal of Nutrition*, Vol 64(1), 1990, pp. 13–22

84 L. J. Whalley *et al.*, 'Cognitive aging, childhood intelligence, and the use of food supplements: Possible involvement of n-3 fatty acids', *American Journal of Clinical Nutrition*, Vol 80(6), 2004, pp. 1650–7

85 W. Snowden, 'Evidence from an analysis of 2000 errors and omissions made in IQ tests by a small sample of schoolchildren, undergoing vitamin and mineral supplementation, that speed of processing is an important factor in IQ performance', *Personality & Individual Differences*, Vol 22(1), Jan 1997, pp.131–4.

86 J. Penland, *Zinc affects cognition and psychosocial function of middle-school children*, Experimental Biology conference, San Diego, April 4, 2005 (pending publication)

87 D. Benton *et al.*, 'Thiamine supplementation mood and cognitive functioning', *Psychopharmacology* (Berl), Vol 129(1), 1997, pp. 66–71.

88 P. Willatts *et al.*, 'Effect of long-chain polyunsaturated fatty acids in infant formula on problem solving at 10 months of age', *Lancet*, Vol 352(9129), 1998, pp. 688–91

89 C. Agostoni *et al.*, 'Developmental quotient at 24 months and fatty acid composition of diet in early infancy: A follow up study', *Archives of Disease in Childhood*, Vol 76(5), 1997, pp. 421–4

90 Jensen *et al.*, 'Effects of maternal docosahexaenoic acid intake on visual function and neurodevelopment in breastfed term infants', *American Journal of Clinical Nutrition*, Vol 82(1), 2005, pp. 125–32

91   I. B. Helland *et al*, 'Maternal Supplementation With Very-Long-Chain n-3 Fatty Acids During Pregnancy and Lactation Augments Children's IQ at 4 Years of Age', *Pediatrics*, Vol. 111(1), pp. e39–e44 (2003)

92   A. Ghys *et al.*, 'Red blood cell and plasma phospholipid arachidonic and docosahexaenoic acid levels at birth and cognitive development at 4 years of age', *Early Human Development*, Vol 69(1–2), October 2002, pp. 83–90

93   L. Horwood and D. M. Fergusson, 'Breastfeeding and later cognitive and academic outcomes', *Pediatrics*, Vol 101, 1998, pp. 1–13

94   C. Lanting *et al.*, 'Neurological differences between 9–year-old children fed breast-milk or formula-milk as babies' *Lancet*, Vol 344(13), 1994, pp. 9–22

95   D. Benton *et al.*, 'Mild hypoglycaemia and questionnaire measures of aggression', *Biological Psychology*, Vol 14(1–2), 1982, pp. 129–35

96   M. Colgan and L. Colgan, 'Do nutrient supplements and dietary changes affect learning and emotional reactions of children with learning difficulties?', *Nutritional Health*, 1984

97   J. Goldman *et al.*, 'Behavioural effects of sucrose on preschool children', *Journal of Abnormal Child Psychology*, Vol 14(4), 1986, pp. 565–77

98   M. Lester *et al.*, 'Refined carbohydrate intake, hair cadmium levels and cognitive functioning in chldren', *Nutrition and Behaviour*, Vol 1, 1982, pp. 3–13

99   S. Schoenthaler *et al.*, 'The impact of a low food additive and sucrose diet on academic performance in 803 New York City public schools', *International Journal of Biosocial Research*, Vol 8(2), 1986, pp. 185–95

100 C. C. Ani and S. M. Grantham-McGregor, 'The effects of breakfast on children's educational performance, attendance and classroom behaviour', in N. Donovan and C. Street (eds), *Fit for School: How breakfast clubs meet health, education and childcare needs*, New Policy Institute, 1999, pp. 14–22, and J. L. Brown, 'New findings about child nutrition and cognitive development', in the same publication, pp. 36–44; and C. Michaud *et al.*, 'Effects of breakfast-size on short-term memory, concentration, mood and blood glucose', *Journal of Adolescent Health*, Vol 12, 1991, pp. 53–7

101 J. P. Jones, H. S. Swartzwelder *et al.*, 'Choline availability to the developing rat fetus alters adult hippocampal long-term potentiation', *Brain Research. Developmental Brain Research*, Vol 118(1–2), 1999, pp. 159–67

102 S. L. Ladd *et al.*, 'Effect of phosphatidylcholine on explicit memory', *Clinical Neuropharmacology*, Vol 16(6), 1993, pp. 540–9

103 *www.autismwebsite.com/ari/treatment/form34q.htm*

104 Judy Shabert *et al.*, *The Ultimate Nutrient – Glutamine*, Avery Publications, 1990

105 T. Ziegler *et al.*, 'Safety and metabolic effects of L-glutamine administration in humans', *Journal of Parenteral and Enteral Nutrition*, Vol 14(4supp), 1990, pp. 137S-146S

106 B. Gesch, 'Influence of supplementary vitamins, minerals and essential fats on the antisocial behaviour of young adult prisoners', *British Journal of Psychiatry*, Vol 181, 2002, pp. 22–8

107 J. R. Hibbeln, 'Fish consumption and major depression', *Lancet*, Vol 351, 1998, pp. 1213

108 B. Nemets *et al.*, 'Addition of omega-3 fatty acid to maintenance medication treatment for recurrent unipolar depressive disorder', *American Journal of Psychiatry*, vol 159, 2002, pp. 477–9

109 B. Puri *et al.*, 'Eicosapentaenoic acid in treatment-resistant depression', *Archives of General Psychiatry*, Vol 59(1), 2002, Letters to the Editor

110 K. A. Smith *et al.*, 'Relapse of depression after rapid depletion of tryptophan', *Lancet*, Vol 349, 1997, pp. 915–19

111 E. Turner *et al.*, 'Serotoninalacarte: Supplementation with the serotonin precursor 5–hydroxytryptophan', *Pharmacology and Therapeutics*, 2005 Jul 13 [Epub ahead of print]

112 H. Cass, 'SAMe – the master tuner supplement for the 21st century', published on www.naturallyhigh.co.uk, 2001

113 B. L. Kagan *et al.*, 'Oral S-adenosylmethionine in depression: A randomized, double-blind, placebo-controlled trial', *American Journal of Psychiatry*, Vol 147(5), 1990, pp. 591–5.

114 P. G. Janicak *et al.*, 'Parenteral S-adenosyl-methionine (SAMe) in depression: Literature review and preliminary data', *Psychopharmacology Bulletin*, Vol 25(2), 1989, pp. 238–42.

115 A. Richardson, 'Fatty acids in dyslexia, dyspraxia, ADHD and the autistic spectrum', *The Nutrition Practitioner*, Vol 3(3), 2001, pp. 18–24

116 A. J. Richardson and J. Wilmer, *Association between fatty acid symptoms and dyslexic and ADHD characteristics in normal college students*, paper given at British Dyslexia Association International Conference, University of York, April 2001

117 M. H. Jorgensen *et al.*, 'Is there a relation between docosahexaenoic acid concentration in mothers' milk and visual development in term infants?' *Journal of Pediatric Gastroenterology and Nutrition*, Vol 32, 2001, pp. 293–6

118 A. J. Richardson *et al.*, *Fatty acid deficiency signs predict the severity of reading and related problems in dyslexic children*, paper given at British Dyslexia Association International Conference, 2001

119 C. M. Absolon *et al.*, 'Psychological disturbance in atopic eczema: The extent of the problem in school-aged children', *British Journal of Dermatology*, Vol 137(2), 1997, pp. 241–5

120 A. J. Richardson *et al.*, 'Abnormal cerebral phospholipid metabolism in dyslexia indicated by phosphorus-31 magnetic resonance spectroscopy', *NMR in Biomedicine*, Vol 10, 1997, pp. 309–14

121 B. J. Stordy, 'Dyslexia, attention deficit hyperactivity disorder, dyspraxia – do fatty acids help?', *Dyslexia Review*, Vol 9(2), 1997, pp. 1–3

122 B. J. Stordy, 'Benefit of decosahexanoic acid supplements to dark adaptation in dyslexia', *Lancet*, Vol 346, 1995, p. 385

123 I. D. Capel *et al.*, 'Comparison of concentrations of some trace, bulk, and toxic metals in the hair of normal and dyslexic children', *Clinical Chemistry*, Vol 27(6), 1981, pp. 879–81

124 R. J. Prinz *et al.*, 'Dietary correlates of hyperactive behaviour in children, *Journal of Consulting and Clinical Psychology*, Vol 48, 1980, pp. 760–69

125 S. J. Schoenthaler *et al.*, 'The effect of randomised vitamin-mineral supplementation on violent and non-violent antisocial behaviour among incarcerated juveniles', *Journal of Nutritional and Environmental Medicine*, 1997

126 L. Langseth and J. Dowd, 'Glucose tolerance and hyperkinesis', *Food and Cosmetic Toxicology*, Vol 16, 1978, p.129

127 I. Colquhon and S. Bunday, 'A lack of essential fats as a possible cause of hyperactivity in children', *Medical Hypotheses,* Vol 7, 1981, pp. 673–9

128 L. J. Stevens *et al.*, 'Essential fat metabolism in boys with attention-deficit hyperactivity disorder', *American Journal of Clinical Nutrition*, Vol 65, 1995, pp. 761–8

129 J. R. Burgess, *ADHD: observational and interventional studies*, NIH workshop on omega-3 EFAs in psychiatric disorder, National Institutes of Health, Bethesda, Maryland, 1998

130 A. J. Richardson *et al.*, *Treatment with highly unsaturated fatty acids can reduce ADHD symptoms in children with specific learning difficulties: a randomised controlled trial*, paper given at British Dyslexia Association International Conference, University of York, April 2001

131 A. Richardson and B. Puri, 'A randomized double-blind, placebo-controlled study of the effects of supplementation with highly unsaturated fatty acids on ADHD-related symptoms in children with specific learning difficulties', *Progress in Neuro-Psychopharmacology and Biological Psychiatry*, Vol 26(2), 2002, pp. 233–9

132 A. Richardson and B. Puri, 'A randomized double-blind, placebo-

controlled study of the effects of supplementation with highly unsaturated fatty acids on ADHD, *Progress in Neuro-Psychopharmacology and Biological Psychiatry*, 2002

133 B. O'Reilly, Hyperactive Children's Support Group Conference, London, June 2001

134 M. D. Boris and F. S. Mandel, 'Foods and additives are common causes of the attention deficit hyperactive disorder in children', *Annals of Allergy*, Vol. 72 (1994), pp. 462–8

135 R. J. Theil, 'Nutrition based interventions for ADD and ADHD', *Townsend Letter for Doctors & Patients*, April 2000, pp. 93–5

136 A. R. Swain *et al.*, 'Salicylates, oligoantigenic diet and behaviour', *Lancet*, Vol. 2(8445), 1985, pp. 41–2

137 B. Starobrat-Hermelin and T. Kozielec, 'The effects of magnesium physiological supplementation on hyperactivity in children with attention deficit hyperactivity disorder (ADHD): Positive response to magnesium oral loading test', *Magnesium Research*, Vol 10(2), 1997, pp. 149–56

138 N. I. Ward, 'Assessment of clinical factors in relation to child hyperactivity', *Journal of Nutritional and Environmental Medicine*, Vol 7, 1997, pp. 333–342

139 N. I. Ward, 'Hyperactivity and a previous history of antibiotic usage', *Nutrition Practitioner*, Vol 3(3), 2001, p. 12

140 S. J. Schoenthaler *et al.*, 'The effect of randomised vitamin-mineral supplementation on violent and non-violent antisocial behaviour among incarcerated juveniles', *Journal of Nutritional and Environmental Medicine*, Vol 7, 1997, pp. 343–52

141 N. D. Volkow *et al.*, 'Therapeutic doses of oral methylphenidate significantly increase extracellular dopamine in the human brain', *Journal of Neuroscience*, Vol 21(RC121), 2001, pp. 1–5

142 S. Chaplin, *The Prescriber*, 5 August 2005, www.escriber.com

143 Dr Joan Baizer of the State University of New York at Buffalo at the Annual Meeting of the Society for Neuroscience, 11 November 2001

144 See www.blockcenter.com/articles2/ritalin_dea.htm and R. D. Ciaranello, 'Attention deficit-hyperactivity disorder and resistance to thyroid hormone-a new idea?', *New England Journal of Medicine*, Vol 328(14), 1993, pp. 1038–9

145 National Institutes of Health, *NIH Consensus Statement: Diagnosis and Treatment of Attention Deficit Hyperactivity Disorder (ADHD)*, NIH, 1998

146 N. Lambert and C. Hartsough, 'Prospective study of tobacco smoking and substance dependencies among samples of ADHD and non-ADHD participants,' *Journal of Learning Disabilities*, Vol 31, 1998, pp. 533–44

147 See the Optimal Wellness Centre website www.mercola. com/2001/jan/7/lendon_smith.htm, and www.smithsez.com/ADHDandADD.html

148 K. Blum and J. Holder, *The Reward Deficiency Syndrome*, American College of Addictionology and Compulsive Disorders, Amereol Ltd, 2002

149 N. D. Volkow *et al.*, 'Therapeutic doses of oral methylphenidate significantly increase extracellular dopamine in the human brain', *Journal of Neuroscience*, 2001

150 R. Huff, *US State Department of Developmental Services Report on Autism*, 1999

151 B. Rimland *et al.*, 'The effect of high doses of vitamin B6 on autistic children: A double-blind crossover study', *American Journal of Psychiatry*, Vol 135(4), 1978, pp. 472–5

152 S. I. Pfeiffer *et al.*, 'Efficacy of vitamin B6 and magnesium in the treatment of autism: A methodology review and summary of outcomes', *Journal of Autism and Developmental Disorders*, Vol 25(5), 1995, pp. 481–93

153 J. Martineau *et al.*, 'Vitamin B6, magnesium, and combined B6–Mg: Therapeutic effects in childhood autism', *Biological Psychiatry*, Vol 20(5), 1985, pp. 467–78

154 S. Vancassel *et al.*, 'Plasma fatty acid levels in autistic children', *Prostaglandins Leukotrienes and Essential Fatty Acids*, Vol 65, 2001, pp. 1–7

155 J. G. Bell *et al.*, 'Red blood cell fatty acid compositions in a patient with autism spectrum disorder: a characteristic abnormality in neurodevelopmental disorders?', *Prostaglandins Leukotrienes and Essential Fatty Acids*, Vol 63(1–2), 2000, pp. 21–5

156 J. G. Bell, *Fatty acid deficiency and phospholipase A2 in autistic spectrum disorders*, workshop report, St Anne's College, Oxford, September 2001

157 M. Megson, 'Is autism a G-Alpha protein defect reversible with natural vitamin A?', *Medical Hypotheses*, Vol 54(6), 2000, pp. 979–83

158 M. Megson, *The biological basis for perceptual deficits in autism: Vitamin A and G-proteins*, lecture given at Ninth International Symposium on Functional Medicine, May 2002

159 Paul Whiteley, the Sunderland University Autism Unit, 'The Biology of Autism – Unravelled', presentation given at the Autism Unravelled Conference, London, May 2001

160 Paul Whitely *et al.*, 'A gluten free diet as an intervention for autism and associated disorders: Preliminary findings', *Autism: International J of Research and Practice*, Vol 3, 1999, pp. 45–65

161 'Anti-fungal drugs more helpful than Ritalin in autistic children', Letter to the Editor, *Townsend Letter for Doctors and Patients*, April 2001, p. 99

162 A. J. Wakefield *et al.*, 'Enterocolitis in children with developmental disorders', *Am J Gastroenterol*, Vol 95(9), 2000, pp. 2285–95

163 M. A. Brudnak, 'Application of genomeceuticals to the molecular and immunological aspects of autism', *Medical Hypotheses*, Vol 57(2), 2001, pp. 186–91

164 P. Varmanen *et al.*, 'S54X-prolyl dipeptidyl aminopeptidase gene (pepX) is part of the glnRA operon in *Lactobaccilus rhamnosus*', *Journal of Bacteriology*, Vol 182(1), 2000, pp. 146–54

165 Paul Whitely *et al.*, 'A gluten free diet as an intervention for autism and associated disorders: Preliminary findings', *Autism: International Journal of Research and Practice*, 1999

166 J. Robert Cade, University of Florida Department of Medicine and Physiology, at www.panix.com/~paleodiet/autism/cadelet.txt

167 M. Ash and E. Gilmore, *Modifying autism through functional nutrition*, paper given at Allergy Research Group conference, London, January 2001

168 Dr Rosemary Waring, University of Birmingham School of Biosciences, 'Sulphate, sulphation and gut permeability: are cytokines involved?', Autism Unravelled Conference Proceedings, London, 11th May, 2001

169 A. J. Wakefield *et al.*, 'Ileal-lymphoid hyperplasia, non-specific colitis, and pervasive developmental disorder in children', *Lancet*, Vol 351, 1998, pp. 637–41

170 Andrew Wakefield, speaking at the Allergy Research Foundation conference, November 1999

171 F. E. Yazbak, 'Autism – is there a vaccine connection?', see www.autisme.net/Yazbak1.htm

172 B. Rimland, *Journal of Nutritional and Environmental Medicine*, Vol 10, 2000, pp. 267–9

173 Ibid. See also Ashcraft & Gerel (law firm), 'Autism caused by childhood vaccinations containing Thimerosal or mercury', at www.ashcraftandgerel.com/thimerosal.html

174 B. Rimland, 'Parents' ratings of the effectiveness of drugs and nutrients', *Autism Research Review International*, Vol 8, October 1994

175 D. B. Smith and E. Obbens, 'Antifolate-antiepileptic relationships', in M. I. Botez and E. H. Reynolds, eds, *Folic Acid in Neurology, Psychiatry and Internal Medicine*, Raven Press (1979)

176 F. B. Gibberd *et al.*, 'The influence of folic acid on the frequency of epileptic attacks', *European Journal of Clinical Pharmacology*, Vol 19(1), 1981, pp. 57–60

177 See ref 175 Smith.

178 M. Nakazawa, 'High dose vitamin B6 therapy in infantile spasms – the effect of adverse reactions', *Brain and Development*, Vol 5(2), 1983, p. 193

179 J. Pietz *et al.*, 'Treatment of infantile spasms with high-dosage vitamin B6', *Epilepsia*, Vol 34(4), 1993, pp. 757–63.

180 A. Sohler and C. Pfeiffer, 'A direct method for the determination of managanese in whole blood: patients with seizure activity have low blood levels', *Journal of Orthomolecular Psychiatry*, Vol 12, 1983, pp. 215–34

181 C. L. Dupont and Y. Tanaka, 'Blood manganese levels in children with convulsive disorder', *Biochemical Medicine*, Vol 33(2), 1985, pp. 246–55

182 P. S. Papavasiliou *et al.*, 'Seizure disorders and trace metals: Manganese tissue levels in treated epileptics', *Neurology*, Vol 29, 1979, p.1466

183 Y. Tanaka, 'Low manganese level may trigger epilepsy', *JAMA – Journal of the American Medical Association*, Vol 238, 1977, p. 1805

184 C. Pfeiffer *et al.*, 'Zinc and manganese in the schizophrenias', *Journal of Orthomolecular Psychiatry*, Vol 12, 1983, pp. 215–34

185 Y. Shoji, 'Serum magnesium and zinc in epileptic children', *Brain and Development*, Vol 5(2), 1983, p. 200

186 S. K. Gupta *et al.*, 'Serum magnesium levels in idiopathic epilepsy', *Journal of the Association of Physicians of India*, Vol 42(6), 1994, pp. 456–7

187 L. F. Gorges *et al.*, 'Effect of magnesium on epileptic foci', *Epilepsia*, Vol 19(1), 1978, pp. 81–91

188 *Pediatria Romania*, Vol 31(4), 1982, pp. 343–7

189 C. L. Zhang *et al.*, 'Paroxysmal epileptiform discharges in temporal lobe slices after prolonged exposure to low magnesium are resistant to clinically used anticonvulsants', *Epilepsy Research*, Vol 20(2), 1995, pp. 105–11

190 Y. Shoji, 'Serum magnesium and zinc in epileptic children', *Journal of Orthomolecular Psychiatry*, 1983

191 A. Barbeau *et al.*, 'Zinc, taurine and epilepsy', *Archives of Neurology*, Vol 30, 1974, pp. 52–8

192 M. I. Botez *et al.*, 'Thiamine and folate treatment of chronic epileptic patients: A controlled study with the Wechsler IQ scale', *Epilepsy Research*, Vol 16(2), 1993, pp. 157–63, and A. Keyser, 'Epileptic manifestations and vitamin B1 deficiency', *European Neurology*, Vol 31(3), 1991, pp. 121–5

193 V. T. Ramaeckers, 'Selenium deficiency triggering intractable seizures', *Neuropediatrics*, Vol 25(4), 1994, pp. 217–23

194 I. R. Tupeev, 'The antioxidant system in the dynamic combined treatment of epilepsy patients with traditional anticonvulsant preparations

and an antioxidant – alpha-tocopherol', *Biulleten Eksperimentalnoi Biologii I Meditsiny*, Vol 116(10), 1993, pp. 362–4

195 S.Yehuda, 'Essential fat preparation (SR-3) raises the seizure threshold in rats', *European Journal of Pharmacology*, Vol 254(1–2), 1994, pp. 193–8

196 S. Schlanger, M. Shinitzky and D.Yam, 'Diet enriched with omega-3 fatty acids alleviates convulsion symptoms in epilepsy patients', *Epilepsia*, Vol 43(1), 2002, pp. 103–4

197 E. S. Roach *et al.*, 'N,N-dimethylglycine for epilepsy', Letter to the Editor, *New England Journal of Medicine*, Vol 307, 1982, pp. 1081–2

198 R. Huxtable *et al.*, 'The prolonged anticonvulsant action of taurine on genetically determined seizure-susceptibility', *Canadian Journal of Neurological Sciences*, Vol 5, 1978, p. 220

199 D. A. Richards *et al.*, 'Extracellular GABA in the ventrolateral thalamus of rats exhibiting spontaneous absence epilepsy: A microdialysis study', *Journal of Neurochemistry*, Vol 65(4), 1995, pp. 1674–80

200 J. Schmidt, 'Comparative studies on the anti-convulsant effectiveness of nootropic drugs in kindled rats', *Biomedica Biochimica Acta*, Vol 49(5), 1990, pp. 413–19

201 B. Gesch, 'Influence of supplementary vitamins, minerals and essential fats on the antisocial behaviour of young adult prisoners', *British Journal of Psychiatry*, Vol 181, 2002, pp. 22–8

202 T. Hamazaki *et al.*, 'The effect of docosahexaenoic acid on aggression in young adults: A placebo-controlled double-blind study', *Journal of Clinical Investigation*, Vol 97, 1996, pp. 1129–33

203 S. J. Schoenthaler *et al.*, 'The effect of randomised vitamin-mineral supplementation on violent and non-violent antisocial behaviour among incarcerated juveniles', *Journal of Nutritional and Environmental Medicine*, Vol 7, 1997, pp. 343–52

204 J. Egger *et al.*, 'Controlled trial of oligoantigenic treatment in the hyperkinetic syndrome', *Lancet*, Vol 1(8428), 1985, pp. 540–5

205 A. G. Schauss and C. E. Simonsen, 'A critical analysis of the diets of chronic juvenile offenders', Part 1, *Journal of Orthomolecular Psychiatry*, Vol. 8(3), 1979, pp. 149–57

206 D. Papalos and J. Papalos, *The Bipolar Child*, Broadway Books, 2000

207 K. Hambidge and A. Silverman, 'Pica with rapid improvement after dietary zinc supplementation', *Archives of Disease in Childhood*, Vol 48, 1973, p. 567

208 R. Bakan, 'The role of zinc in anorexia nervosa: Etiology and treatment', *Medical Hypotheses*, Vol 5(7), 1979, pp. 731–6

209 D. Horrobin and S. C. Cunnane, 'Interactions between zinc, essential fatty acids and prostaglandins: Relevance to acrodermatitis enteropatica, total parenteral nutrition, and glucagonoma syndrome,

diabetes, anorexia nervosa, and sickle cell anemia', *Medical Hypotheses*, Vol 6, 1980, pp. 277–96

210 R. C. Casper and A. S. Prasad, 1980, later confirmed by L. Humphries *et al.*, 'Zinc deficiency and eating disorders', *Journal of Clinical Psychiatry*, Vol 50(12), 1980, pp. 456–9

211 P. R. Flanagan, 'A model to produce pure zinc deficiency in rats and its use to demonstrate that dietary phytate increases the excretion of endogenous zinc', *Journal of Nutrition*, Vol 114, 1984, pp. 493–502, and A. Grider *et al.*, 'Age-dependent influence of dietary zinc restriction on short-term memory in male rats', *Physiology and Behaviour*, Vol 72(3), 2001, pp. 339–48

212 A. Arcasoy *et al.*, 'Ultrastructural changes in the mucosa of the small intestine in patients with geophagia (Prasad's syndrome)', *Journal of Pediatric Gastroenterology and Nutrition*, Vol 11(2), 1990, pp. 279–82

213 D. Bryce-Smith and R. I. Simpson, 'Case of anorexia nervosa responding to zinc sulphate', *Lancet*, Vol 2(8398), 1984, p. 350

214 Katz *et al.*, *J Adol Health Care*, Vol 8, 1987, pp. 400–6

215 L. Humphries *et al.*, 'Zinc deficiency and eating disorders', *Journal of Clinical Psychiatry*, 1989

216 N. F. Shay and H. F. Mangian, 'Neurobiology of zinc-influenced eating behavior', *Journal of Nutrition*, Vol 130(5S Suppl), 2000, pp. 1493S-9S

217 R. Bakan *et al.*, 'Dietary zinc intake of vegetarian and non-vegetarian patients with anorexia nervosa', *International Journal of Eating Disorders*, Vol 13(2), 1993, pp. 229–33

218 F. Askenazy *et al.*, 'Whole blood serotonin content, tryptophan concentrations, and impulsivity in anorexia nervosa', *Biological Psychiatry*, Vol 43(3), 1998, pp. 188–95

219 A. Favaro, 'Tryptophan levels, excessive exercise, and nutritional status in anorexia nervosa', *Psychosomatic Medicine*, Vol 62(4), 2000, pp. 535–8

220 P. J. Cowen and K. A. Smith, 'Serotonin, dieting, and bulimia nervosa', *Advances in Experimental Medicine and Biology*, Vol 467, 1999, pp. 101–4.

221 Y. Harrison and J. A. Horne, 'Sleep deprivation affects speech', *Sleep*, Vol 20(10), 1997, pp. 871–7

222 L. Ozturk *et al.*, 'Effects of 48 hours sleep deprivation on human immune profile', *Sleep Res Online*, Vol 2(4), 1999, pp. 107–11

223 Judith Owens *et al.*, 'Television-viewing habits and sleep disturbance in school children', *Pediatrics*, Vol 104(3), 1999, pp. 27

224 M. G. Smits *et al.*, 'Melatonin for chronic sleep onset insomnia in children: A randomized placebo-controlled trial', *Journal of Child Neurology*, Vol 16(2), 2001, pp. 86–92

225 E. J. Pavonen *et al.*, 'Effectiveness of melatonin in the treatment of

sleep disturbances in children with Asperger disorder', *Journal of Child and Adolescent Psychopharmacology*, Vol 13(1), 2003, pp. 83–95

226 American Dietetic Association, 'Promotion of breastfeeding', *Journal of American Dietetic Association*, no. 97, 1997, pp. 662–6

227 M. Martin, 'Is DHA the secret of breast milk's success?' *WorldNetDaily.com*, 2002

228 E. L. Mortensen *et al.*, 'The association between duration of breast-feeding and adult intelligence', *JAMA – Journal of the American Medical Association*, Vol 287, 2002, pp. 2365–71

229 F. Martinez, 'Evaluation of plasma tocopherols in relation to hemato-logical indices of Brazilian infants on human milk and cows' milk regime from birth to 1 year of age' *American Journal of Clinical Nutrition*, Vol. 41(3), 1985, pp. 969–74

230 C. Kunz, *International Journal for Vitamin & Nutrient Research*, Vol. 54(141), 1984

231 W. Craig, *Nutrition Reports International*, Vol 30(4), 1984, p. 1003

232 J. Armstrong, J. J. Reilly and the Child Health Information Team, 'Breastfeeding and lowering the risk of childhood obesity', *Lancet*, Vol 359(9322), 2002, pp. 2003–4

233 N. I. Ward, 'Hyperactivity and a previous history of antibiotic usage', *Nutrition Practitioner*, Vol 3(3), 2001, p. 12

234 N. I. Ward, 'Assessment of clinical factors in relation to child hyperac-tivity', *Journal of Nutritional and Environmental Medicine*, Vol 7, 1997, pp. 333–42

235 R. L. William *et al.*, 'Use of antibiotics in preventing recurrent acute otitis media and in treating otitis media with effusion', *JAMA – Journal of the American Medical Association*, Vol 270, 1993, pp. 1344–51

236 J. Braly and R. Hoggan, *Dangerous Grains*, Avery, 2002, p. 24

RECOMMENDED READING

Child, S., *An A-Z of Child Health: A Nutritional Approach*, Argyll, 2002

Holford, P., *The New Optimum Nutrition Bible,* Piatkus, 2005

Holford, P. and Lawson, S., *Optimum Nutrition Before During and After Pregnancy*, Piatkus, 2004

Holford, P. and Braly, J., *Hidden Food Allergies*, Piatkus, 2005

Holford, P., *The Holford Low-GL Diet*, Piatkus, 2004

Holford, P. and McDonald Joyce, F., *The Holford Low-GL Diet Cookbook*, Piatkus, 2005

Holford, P., and Ridgeway, J. *The Optimum Nutrition Cookbook*, Piatkus, 2000

Wigmore, A., *The Sprouting Book*, Avery, 1986

RESOURCES

Mind and nutrition

The Brain Bio Centre is a London-based treatment centre founded by Patrick Holford that puts the optimum nutrition approach into practice for people with mental health problems, including learning difficulties, dyslexia, ADHD, autism, Alzheimer's, dementia, memory loss, depression, anxiety and schizophrenia.

For more information, visit www.brainbiocentre.com or call 020 8871 9261. *8332 9600*

The Institute for Optimum Nutrition (ION) offers a three-year foundation degree course in nutritional therapy that includes training in the optimum nutrition approach to mental health. There is a clinic, a list of nutrition practitioners across the UK, an information service and a quarterly journal – *Optimum Nutrition*.

Contact ION at Avalon House, 72 Lower Mortlake Road, Richmond TW9 2JY, UK, or call 020 8877 9993 or visit www.ion.ac.uk.

To find a nutritional therapist near you who we recommend, visit www.patrickholford.com and click on 'consultations'.

Food for the Brain is an educational charity to promote the link between optimum nutrition and mental health. The Food for the Brain Schools Campaign also gives advice to schools and parents on how to make kids smarter by improving the quality of food in and outside of school.

Visit www.foodforthebrain.org for further information.

Food and Behaviour Research is a charitable organisation dedicated both to advancing scientific research into the links between nutrition and human behaviour and to making the findings from such research available to the widest possible audience.

They have an excellent website and a free e-news service. Sign up at www.fabresearch.org.

The Food and Mood Project aims to empower individuals to explore the relationship between diet, nutrition and emotional and mental health, and to share this information with others. They have a quarterly newsletter, put on conferences and work closely with Mind to help improve awareness of the nutrition link to mental health problems.

For more information, visit www.foodandmood.org.

Mental health – general

ChildLine (800 1111) is a free helpline for children and young people in the UK, who can call 24 hours a day, every day of the year, to talk to counsellors about any problem.

The British Association for Counselling and Psychotherapy has an online directory of suitably qualified therapists. Visit their website at www.bacp.co.uk.

Mental Health Foundation is an organisation that provides all sorts of useful information on mental health, and keeps a very comprehensive list of mental health organisations. Contact the UK office of the Mental Health Foundation at 7th Floor, 83 Victoria Street, London SW1H 0HW, UK, or call their helpline on 020 7802 0302, or visit www.mentalhealth.org.uk.

Mind is the leading mental health charity in England and Wales, working for a better life for everyone with experience of mental distress. Mind does this by advancing the views, needs and ambitions of people with experience of mental distress; promoting inclusion by challenging discrimination; influencing policy through campaigning and education; inspiring the development of quality services, which reflect expressed need and diversity; and achieving equal civil and legal rights through campaigning and education.

Their website www.mind.org.uk is full of useful information, including details on your nearest local association. Or contact Mind at Granta House, Broadway, London E15, UK, or call 020 8215 2499.

Specific conditions

ADHD/Hyperactivity

The Hyperactive Children's Support Group (HACSG) is a UK-based charity organisation that offers support and information to parents and professionals who wish to pursue a drug-free approach to treating ADHD. They help and support hyperactive children and their parents, conduct research, promote investigation into the incidence of hyperactivity in the UK, investigate its causes and treatments, and spread information concerning the condition. There are some local groups in the UK which have been started by the parents of hyperactive children. There are also contact parents who have offered to help newly joined members in their locality.

Contact HACSG at 71 Whyke Lane, Chichester, West Sussex P019 2PD, UK, for all information, diet booklets, articles and general requests (enclose a stamped SAE). Or call 01243 551313, or visit www.hacsg.org.uk.

Allergies

Action Against Allergy (AAA) is a national charity founded by a multi-allergy sufferer some 30 years ago. AAA provides information across the whole spectrum of allergies and allergy-related illness. Specialist referral contacts and wide-ranging advisory leaflets are available. Membership gives access to the Talkline support network and free *Allergy Newsletter*. Call 020 8892 2711/4949, email AAA@actionagainstallergy.freeserve.co.uk or visit actionagainstallergy.co.uk, where you can order online.

Autism

The National Autistic Society UK was founded in 1962 by parents frustrated by the lack of provision and support for children with autism and their carers, with the aim of encouraging a better understanding of autism and to pioneer specialist services for people with autism and those who care for them.

Contact the National Autistic Society UK at 393 City Road, London EC1V 1NG, UK, or call 020 7833 2299, or visit www.nas.org.uk.

Autism Research Institute (ARI), founded by Bernard Rimland PhD, is the hub of a worldwide network of parents and professionals concerned with autism. The only organisation of its kind, ARI was founded in 1967 to conduct and foster scientific research designed to improve the methods of diagnosing, treating and preventing autism. ARI also disseminates research findings to parents and others all over the world who are seeking help. The ARI data bank, the world's largest, contains nearly 25,000 detailed case histories of autistic children from over 60 countries.

Contact ARI at 4182 Adams Avenue, San Diego, California 92116, US, or visit www.autism.com/ari.

Autism Unravelled is a registered UK charity providing carers, sufferers and professionals with fundamental, impartial and up-to-date information on known, current and theoretical research into the causes and treatments of autistic spectrum disorders.

Visit www.autism-unravelled.com for further information.

Dyslexia

The British Dyslexia Association offers advice, information and help to families, professionals and dyslexic individuals, and is working to raise awareness and understanding of dyslexia, and to effect change.

Contact the British Dyslexia Association at 98 London Road, Reading, RG1 5AU, UK, or call their helpline 0118 966 8271, or visit www.bda-dyslexia.org.uk.

The Dyslexia Institute is an educational charity, founded in 1972, for the assessment and teaching of people with dyslexia and for the training of teachers. They can assess your child using a psychological test. Most schools also offer testing as well as providing special needs teachers to help your child with their areas of difficulties. This assessment is necessary for extra time allowance in exams.

Contact the Dyslexia Institute at 133 Gresham Rd, Staines, Middlesex TW18 2AJ, UK, or call 01784 463 851, or visit www.dyslexia-inst.org.uk.

The Bates Association for Vision Education for information on natural vision improvement and a list of qualified teachers visit www.seeing.org.

Eating disorders

Eating Disorders Association provides help and support for people affected by eating disorders, particularly anorexia nervosa, bulimia and binge eating.

Call their helpline 01603 621414 or visit www.edauk.com.

Laboratory testing

Food allergy (IgG ELISA) and homocysteine testing is available through York Test Laboratories, using a home test kit where you can take your own pinprick blood sample and return it to the lab for analysis.

Contact FREEPOST NEA5 243 York YO19 5ZZ, freephone 0800 0746185 or visit www.yorktest.com.

Hair mineral analyses are available from Trace Elements, Inc. (US), a leading laboratory for hair mineral analysis for healthcare professionals worldwide.

Visit www.traceelements.com for more details or contact the UK agent Mineral Check at 62 Cross Keys, Bearsted, Maidstone, Kent ME14 4HR, UK. Or call 01622 630044, or visit www.mineralcheck.com.

Biolab carry out blood tests for essential fats, urine tests for pyroluria, chemical sensitivity panels, toxic element screens, and more. Only available through qualified practitioners.

Contact Biolab at The Stone House, 9 Weymouth Street, London W1W 6DB, UK, or call 020 7636 5959, or visit www.biolab.co.uk.

European Laboratory of Nutrients (ELN) provide a wide range of biochemical tests including mineral profiles, fatty acid profile, thyroid function test, hormone profiles and neurotransmitter tests. European Laboratory of Nutrients, Regulierenring 9, 3981 LA Bunnik, The Netherlands. Phone: 011–31–(0)30–287–1492.

PRODUCT AND SUPPLEMENT DIRECTORY

Supplements

Multivitamin and mineral supplements

The best chewable multivitamin, based on optimum nutrition
levels, is Higher Nature's Dinochews. For older children who can
swallow capsules, Higher Nature's Advanced Optimum Nutrition
Formula is ideal. Very young children can take Ola Loa (from
www.drinkyourvitamins.com) – a multi in a sachet that is mixed
with water to make a pleasant-tasting slightly effervescent drink.
Calma-C from Higher Nature provides additional calcium and
magnesium for growing children as a pleasant-tasting drink.

Biocare make an excellent range of liquid mineral and vitamin
products. These can be added in drop form to other drinks and
food. In addition, Biocare make a couple of vitamin C powder
products which provide additional minerals and can also be added
to drinks or food.

Essential fats and fish oil supplements

The most important omega-3 fats are DHA and EPA, the richest
source being cod liver oil. The most important omega-6 fat is
GLA, the richest source being borage (also known as starflower)
oil. Our favourite supplement is Higher Nature's Essential Omegas,
which provides a highly concentrated mix of EPA, DHA and
GLA. Higher Nature also make Smartfish, a flavoured fish oil gel in
a sachet that kids can squeeze into their mouths.

Seven Seas makes a very good Extra High Strength Cod Liver Oil, which also contains vitamin A. Nutri's Eskimo-3 or Eskimo for Kids are very good sources of EPA and DHA – the Kids version being a non-fishy-tasting liquid, while the original is a fairly neutral unflavoured version.

Vegetarian options do not provide EPA and DHA directly, only the precursors – so they're not our first choice for these omega-3s. But if you want to go for this, choose an Omega Nutrition product from Higher Nature – either oil, flavoured oil or capsules. If you choose a flavoured oil and your child has food allergies, check the list of ingredients carefully.

Probiotics

We recommend Higher Nature's Acidobifidus powder or Biocare's Strawberry or Banana Acidophilus, a powder to be added to food or drink. Infants need a particular age-appropriate strain of probiotic available from Biocare called Bifidobacterium Infantis. Older children who can swallow capsules can take Biocare's Bio-Acidophilus. *Saccharomyces boulardii*, while not strictly a probiotic, plays a very important role in improving gut immunity. This product is only available in the UK through a nutritional therapist. Visit www.patrickholford.com and click on 'consultations' to find a nutritionist in your area.

Homocysteine-lowering nutrients

Several companies produce good homocysteine-lowering formulations. Higher Nature makes H-Factors, and Solgar, Homocysteine Modulators. H-Factors has the advantage of containing B12 in the form of methylcobalamin, which is the most effective form. Both of these supplements come in tablet form only, which will need to be ground in a coffee grinder and mixed into food. Homocysteine-lowering nutrients are usually only needed for a few weeks or months at the most.

Brain support and phospholipid supplements

Additional brain nutrients include phospholipids such as phosphatidyl choline and phosphatidyl serine, and pyroglutamate and DMAE. Phosphatidyl choline (PC) can be found in lecithin granules which are a pleasant-tasting addition to breakfast. Higher Nature's High PC Lecithin Granules contain 30 per cent more PC than other lecithins. Higher Nature's Advanced Brain Food Formula contains a blend of these brain support nutrients, plus some ginkgo.

Company directory

In the UK

The following companies produce good-quality supplements that are widely available in the UK.

Health Products for Life is an online shop that stocks most of the supplements and other products mentioned above, including Xylosweet (the sugar substitute xylitol).

You can order from them directly from the website www.healthproductsforlife.com or by telephone on 020 8874 8038.

Higher Nature produces an extensive range of nutritional and herbal supplements, including Get Up & Go, which are available in all good health food shops and by mail order.

Call 0845 3300012 for your nearest stockist, or 01435 882880 for a full-colour catalogue and free newsletter. Visit www.higher-nature.co.uk for information and to place postal orders, or write to them at Burwash Common, East Sussex TN19 7LX, UK, or email sales@higher-nature.co.uk.

Biocare produce a wide range of nutritional and herbal supplements, including an excellent children's range, which are available in any good health food shop. For your nearest supplier, call 0121 433 3727 or visit www.biocare.co.uk.

Seven Seas specialise in cod liver oil, rich in omega-3 fats. Their products are widely available in health food stores, supermarkets and pharmacies, or visit www.seven-seas.ltd.uk.

Solgar produce a wide range of nutritional and herbal supplements available in any good health food shop. For your nearest supplier, visit www.solgar.co.uk or call 01442 890355.

In other regions

South Africa   Bioharmony produce a wide range of products in South Africa and other African countries. For details of your nearest supplier contact 0860 888 339 or visit www.bioharmony.co.za.

Australia   Solgar supplements are available in Australia. Contact Solgar on 1800 029 871 (free call) for your nearest supplier, or visit www.solgar.com.au. Another good brand is Blackmores.

New Zealand   Higher Nature products are available in New Zealand. Contact Aurora Natural Therapies, 445 Dillons Point Road, RD3, Blenheim, Marlborough, New Zealand, or call (64) 3578 1236/(64) 27449 8573, or visit www.aurora.org.nz.

Singapore   Higher Nature and Solgar products are available in Singapore. Please contact Essential Living on 6276 1380 for your nearest supplier or visit www.essliv.com.

£29.99 1 yr
49.99 2 yr

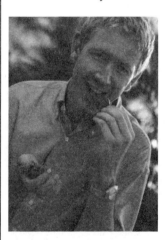

INDEX

Note: page numbers in **bold** refer to illustrations, page numbers in *italics* refer to information contained in tables.

Abolson, Christine 152
acetylcholine 56–7, 62, 72, 122–4, 168
additives (anti-nutrients) 18, 85–92, 235
  and hyperactivity 5, 161
  least harmful 87
  top 20 87–91
adolescents
  aggressive behaviour of 194
  and eating disorders 199, 204
adrenalin 16, 62, 139–44
aggressive behaviour 193–8
  and anti-nutrients 78, 83, 85, 193–4
  and blood sugar balance 24, 195
  and food allergies 93, 197
  minerals for 76, 196
allergens (anti-nutrients) 19, 93–100
allura red (E129) 87
alpha-linolenic acid 47, 48–9, 52
aluminium *79*, 80, 164, 193–4
amaranth (E123) 87
American Journal of Psychiatry 36
amino acids 16–17, 18, 60–1, 63, 65–6,
  141–3
  checking your child's status 61
  deficiencies 60
  and epilepsy 189–91
  essential 63
  excess intake 65
amphetamines 62
  see also Ritalin
anaphylactic shock 89, 90
anger 136
anorexia nervosa 76, 199–207
anthocyanidins 75
anti-fungal agents 181, 184
anti-nutrients 6, 9, 14, 18–19
  additives 5, 18, 85–92, 161, 235
  and ADHD 163–4
  food allergens 19, 93–100
  heavy metals 18, 78–84, *79*, 182–3
antibiotics 99–100, 163, 177, 223, 227

antibodies 95–6, **95–6**
antidepressants 62–3, 135
  natural 143
antioxidants 70, 73–5, **74**, 77
  additives 87, 90
anxiety
  and blood sugar balance 24
  and caffeine 36
  and essential fatty acids 42
  and food allergies 93
  minerals for 76
appetite 203, 205–7
arachidonic acid (AA) 13, 50, 152–3, 159
artificial sweeteners 32, 88, 90
aspartame (E951) 32, 88
Asperger's syndrome 4, 170, 175
asthma 86–91, 220
attention deficit disorder (ADD) 24, 40–1
attention deficit hyperactivity disorder
  (ADHD) 4, 149, **150**, 155–69, 223
  and autism 170, 172, 183
  and bipolar disorder 197, 198
  and blood sugar balance 118, 156–7
  checklist for 156–7
  DMAE for 123
  and epilepsy 185
  essential fats for 42, 49, 152, 156,
    158–60, 162, 225
  and food allergies 93, 94, 97, 156,
    160–2
autism 4, 5, 6–7, 170–92
  digestive problems of 176–8, 181
  early-/late-onset dichotomy 182
  and epilepsy 185–91
  and essential fats 40–1, 172, 173–4
  and food allergies 93–4, 97, 172,
    175–80, **178**, 183, 191
  minerals for 76, 172, 173, 177
  and the MMR vaccine 181–3, 191
  prevalence 171, **171**
  symptoms of 170

Autism Research Unit 176, 178–9
autistic spectrum disorders 170–92

Baizer, Joan 165
Bakan, Rita 202
bananas 21
barbeques 75
barley 97
Bates Method 128
beans 242–3
behaviour 6, 135–45
  assessing your child's 106
  and DMAE 123
  and essential fats 40–1, 42, 48–9
Bell, Gordon 173
Bellanti, Joseph 160–1
Benton, David 2, 23–4, 67, 72, 109
benzoic acid (E210) 88
beta-carotene 75
Biederman, Joseph 197
Bifidobacteria 220
binge eating 200, 201, 207–8
biotin 159
bipolar children 197–8
birth defects 73
blood sugar balance 18, 20–38
  and ADHD 118, 156–7
  and aggressive behaviour 24, 195
  and autism 172
  carbohydrates and 22, 24–30, 117–18
  checking your child's 21–2
  and concentration problems 21, 24,
    117–22
  eating breakfast for 27–8, 34–5, 38,
    119–21, 125
  effects of imbalance 23–4
  and mood 136–7
  process of 22–3
  and sleep problems 209, 211, 212
  steps to 30–7
  vitamins for 72
body–mind connection 11
borage/starflower oil 49, 52
brain 11–19, **15**
  development 12–14, 48
  and gut health 223
Brain Bio Centre 3–4, 20–1, 39, 45,
    93–4, 107, 144, 156, 187, 193–4, 209
brain foods, essential 6, 9–77
  fats 18, 39–54
  phospholipids 18, 55–9
  protein 18, 60–6
  vitamins and minerals 18, 67–77
  see also blood sugar balance

bread 27–8, 240–1
breakfasts
  and blood sugar balance 27–8, 34–5,
    38, 119–21, 125
  clubs 119, 246
  ideas for 240–1, 242
breastfeeding 223, 227
  and intelligence 41–2, 115, 219–20
  and vitamin/mineral intake 69, 220
Breggin, Peter 165
brilliant black BN (E151) 88
British Journal of Psychiatry 137, 194
Bryce-Smith, Derek 203–4
bulimia nervosa 199–203, 205–7
burnout 141
butylated hydroxy-ansole (E320) 88

Cade, Robert 178
cadmium 78, *79*, 80
caffeine 35–7, 38
calcium *70*, 76
  and aggressive behaviour 196
  and sleep problems 209, 211, 214
  sources 225–6, *226*
calcium benzoate (E213) 88
calcium sulphite (E226) 89
carbohydrates
  and blood sugar balance 22, 24–30,
    117–18
  complex 24, **26**, 158
  fast-releasing 24–5, 27
  and fibre 32–3
  food combining 32–3, 38, 158
  refined 18, 22, 24–5, 31–2, 38, 118,
    156–8
  simple 24, **26**
  slow-releasing 25, 27
  sugar family **26**
carcinogens 88–90
case studies
  ADHD 156, 160
  aggressive behaviour 193–4
  autism 171–2, 184–5
  effects of blood sugar balance 20–1
  effects of essential fats 39
  food allergies 93–4
  heavy metal intake 78–9
  IQ boosting food 107
  mood problems 4, 144
  reading/writing problems 4, 127–8
  sleep problems 209
casein 175, 176, 178–80, **178**, 183
cereals 240
cerebral cortex 14–16

cheese 234
chicken nuggets 238–9
chocolate 35–6
choice, children's 230–1
cholesterol 42–3, 53–4, 58
co-enzyme Q 75
coconut oil 243
cod liver oil 132–3, 174, 175
coffee 36, 37
colas 35
colic 220
concentration problems
   and anti-nutrients 78, 85
   and blood sugar balance 21, 24, 117–22
   checking for 105
   essential fatty acids for 42
   vitamins/minerals for 72, 77
Concerta 164
constipation 93–4, 156
cooking fats/oils 243–4
coordination problems 41, 151, 153
   checking for 106
copper 79, 82
   and ADHD 163, 166
   and dyslexia/dyspraxia 153
   and epilepsy 188
cortisol 212
Cowen, Philip 141, 206
creative thinking 105
cystine 83

dairy foods 234
   allergies to 96–7, 99, 175, 178–80, 183,
      191, 225, 241
   and binge eating 207
   protein content 65
Deaner/Deanol 123, 167
delinquency 76
   see also young offenders
dendrites 16
deoxyribonucleic acid (DNA) 103
depression 4
   amongst young people 135, 136
   and anti-nutrients 78, 85
   and blood sugar balance 24
   and caffeine 36
   and essential fats 40–1
   and food allergies 93
   and protein deficiency 60
   vitamins/minerals for 72, 76
dermatitis/eczema 86, 89, 220
detoxing 180–1
DGLA (dihomogamma-linolenic acid)
   13, 49, 153

digestive health 223
dinners 241–2
DMAE (2-dimethylaminoethanol)
   123–4, 126, 167–8, 190
DMG (di-methyl glycine) 189
docosahexaenoic acid (DHA) 13, 47–9,
   53, 152–3, 159
   and breastfeeding 220
   and intelligence 41, 114–15, 114
   recommended intake 114–15
   sources 50, 51, 52
   supplementation 115, 253
dopamine 16, 62, 139, 168
Down's syndrome 108–9
drinks
   fizzy 35, 118, 121–2, 125
   fruit juice 33–4, 38, 158, 234
   healthy 122
dysbiosis 181
dysgraphia 78–9
dyslexia 128, 149–54, 150
   assessing your child for 128, 131–2,
      150–1
   and autism 170, 172
   and epilepsy 185
   and essential fats 40–1, 49, 115,
      152–4
Dyslexia Institute 151
dyspraxia 149–54, 150
   and autism 170, 172
   and epilepsy 185
   and essential fats 50

E numbers 86, 87–91, 235
eating disorders 24, 199–208
eating out 232
eczema/dermatitis 86, 89, 220
Egger, Joseph 94
eggs 49, 58–9, 96–7, 234
eicosapentaenoic acid (EPA) 13, 47–9,
   152–3, 159
   and autism 174
   and IQ 115
   sources 50, 51, 52
   supplementation 115, 253
elimination and challenge diets 98,
   178–9, 178
emotional eating 230, 231
emotional intelligence (EQ) 41, 104
emphysema 89, 90
endorphins 62
enlightenment 104
enteric nervous system 223
enzymes 103

epilepsy 185–91
temporal lobe 187–8
essential fats 16, 18, 40–52
action in the body 42–4
adding to meals 241
for ADHD 42, 49, 152, 156, 158–60,
162, 225
and aggressive behaviour 195–6
and autism 40–1, 172, 173–4
checking your child's levels of 152
conversion problems 159, 162
deficiency 40–1, 45–7
in the diet 44–50
for dyslexia/dyspraxia 40–1, 49, 115,
152–4
and eating disorders 206, 207
and epilepsy 186, 189
for the eyes 132–3, 152, 153
and intelligence 41–2, 110, 113–15
and learning difficulties 152
for mood 137, 138–9, 144, 145
recommended intake 45–6, **46**, 48
for speech and language delay 39
supplementation *250*, 252–3
see also omega-3 essential fats; omega-6
essential fats
evening primrose oil 49–50, 52, 160
exhaust fumes 73–4
exorphins 176–7, 178, 180, 207
eyes/eyesight 128, 132–4, 151
black and white vision of autism 174–5
essential fats for 132–3, 152, 153
Eysenck, Hans 109

fat, body 23
fat, cooking 243–4
fat, dietary 39–54
to avoid/limit 18, 44–5, 52–4
brain's need for 12–13
checking your child's levels of 21–2
cholesterol 42–3, 53–4, 58
hydrogenated 52, 233
monounsaturated 42, 53
polyunsaturated 46
saturated 42, 45, 46, **46**, 53
trans fats 45, 52–3
types of 13
see also essential fats
'fat free' products 236–7
fatigue 24, 40–1, 93
Feingold diet 161–2
'few foods' diet 5
fibre 25, 32–3
fish fingers 238–9

fish oils 52, 54, 115
cod liver oil 132–3, 174, 175
for the eyes 132–3
and IQ 2
for speech and language delay 39
vitamin A content 133–4
fish, oily 47–8, 49, 50, 51, 54
DHA content 114–15, *114*
and IQ 114
mercury content 81, *81–2*, 114
protein content *64*
fits 170, 185–91
fizzy drinks 35, 118, 121–2, 125
flavour enhancers 89, 96
flaxseed oil 48, 51
flaxseeds 48, 50
flower foods 64
foetal development 12–14, 48
folic acid *70*, 72–3, 112, 137, 186
food allergies 19, 93–100, **95–6**
and ADHD 93, 94, 97, 156, 160–2
and aggressive behaviour 93, 193–4, 197
and autism 93–4, 97, 172, 175–80, **178**,
183, 191
and breastfeeding 220
definition 95
immunoglobulin type E 95–6, **95**, 98
immunoglobulin type G 95, **96**, 98
and mood 136
prevention 221–2
and sleep problems 209, 211, 213
symptoms of 93
testing for 93–4, 98–9, 100
top ten allergenic foods 96–7
Food for the Brain Campaign 248, 254–5
food colourings 86–91, 161
food combining 32–3, 38, 158
food diaries 179
food intolerances 95–6
food preparation 239
food sensitivities 95–6
free radicals (oxidants) 73–4, **74**, 77
fructose 25
fruit
dried 25
Glycemic Load *28–9*
most beneficial 121
organic 91–2
sugars of 25, 31–2
fruit juice 33–4, 38, 158, 234
fussy eaters 228–32

gamma-aminobutyric acid (GABA) 61,
62, 124, 190

gamma-linolenic acid (GLA) 49–53, 159, 253
garlic 97
genes 103
Gesch, Bernard 4, 137–8
gliadin 97
Global Developmental Delay 107
glucose tolerance, abnormal 157
glutamine 124–5, 253
L-glutamine 177–8
glutathione 75
gluten allergies 93–4, 96–7, 176–9, **178**, 183, 191
Glycemic Load (GL) 26–30
    of breakfasts 119–20
    of common foods *26–30*
    of fruit juices 34
glycine 88
glycogen 23, 31–2
grains 38, *64*
Grant, Charles 168
grazing 121
growth hormone 212
guarana 35
Guardian (newspaper) 201
Gull, William 201
gut bacteria 177, 181, 220, 223

hair mineral analysis 79, 83, 84, 164
Hamazaki, Tomohito 195
Hambridge, Michael 202
Harrell, Ruth 108–9
Harris, Gillian 224
Hayward, Karen 118
headaches 88–90
hemp seeds 50
hemp-seed oil 52
herbal remedies, for epilepsy 190
Hibbeln, Joseph 138
Hill, Nigel 118
histamine 95
homocysteine levels 5, 144
    and aggressive behaviour 193–4
    and school grades 14
    and vitamin B levels 14, 71
Horrobin, David 203
Hyperactive Children's Support Group 159–60, 161
hyperactivity 4, 5, 6–7, 128
    and anti-nutrients 86, 91
    and blood sugar balance 24
    checklist for 156–7
    and food allergies 93, 94, 97
    minerals for 76

hyperactivity – *contd*
    see also attention deficit hyperactivity disorder
hypoglycaemia 195

IAG 176
immune system 95–6, **95–6**, 210
immunoglobulin type E (IgE) 95–6, **95**, 98
immunoglobulin type G (IgG) 95, **96**, 98–9
immunoglobulin type G (IgG) ELISA test 93–4, 98–9, 100
impulsivity 78, 85
Independent Television (ITV) 4
inflammation 50
information processing, speed of 111–15
Institute for Optimum Nutrition 3, 67, 109, 203
    see also Brain Bio Centre
insulin 22–3
intelligence 2, 104–5
    checking your child's 105–6
    and essential fats 41–2, 110, 113–15
    facets of 41, 104
    vitamins and minerals for 67–8, 69, 108–13, *112–13*
    see also concentration problems; memory problems
intelligence quotient (IQ) 2, 6, 107–16
    and anti-nutrients 78, 82–3, 85, 109
    assessment 105
    and blood sugar balance 23
    and breastfeeding 219–20
    and essential fats 41, 110, 113–15
    non-verbal 109
    vitamins and minerals for 67–8, 69, 108–13, *112–13*
intestinal flora 177, 181, 220, 223
iron 166
isoleucine 205

Journal of the American Medical Association 187, 223

kryptopyrroles 173
Kubala, Albert 108

lactose intolerance 96
Lancet, The (journal) 68, 109
lead *79*, 82
leaky gut syndrome 99, 177, 180
learning difficulties
    and blood sugar balance 24

learning difficulties – *contd*
  DMAE for 123
  essential fats for 42, 48–9, 115, 152
  and food allergies 93
lecithin 58–9, 122, 125, 253
lentils 242–3
light 140–1
linoleic acid 49, 50, 52
lipoic acid 75
liver 180
lunch boxes 246–7
lunches 241–2

magnesium 70, 76
  and ADHD 156, 159, 162, 166, 167
  and aggressive behaviour 196
  and autism 172, 173
  deficiency 39, 107
  and epilepsy 186, 187–8
  for mood 137, 138, 144
  and sleep problems 209, 211, 214
  supplementation 138, 252
manganese 166, 186, 187
Medical Research Council 69
Megson, Mary 174, 175, 183
melatonin 72, 213–15
Mellaril 167
memory problems 6, 122–6
  and anti-nutrients 78, 85
  and blood sugar balance 24
  and caffeine 37
  checking for 105
  and essential fats 40–1
  phospholipids for 56, 57–8
  vitamins/minerals for 72, 77
mental retardation 108–9, 110
mercury 48, 78, 79, 80–1, 114–15, 182–3
metals, toxic 18, 78–84, 79, 182–3
  see also aluminium; copper; mercury
methionine 83
methylation 72, 137
milk 225–6, 231, 234
  allergies to 96–7, 183, 225
  goat's 97, 226
  sheep's 97, 226
mind–body connection 11
minerals 18, 67–9, 70, 75–7
  checking your child's intake 68
  IQ boosting 67–8, 69, 108–13, *113*
  key **70**
  and mood 136
  supplementation 249–53, *250*
  see also multivitamins and minerals;
    specific minerals

MMR (measles, mumps, rubella) vaccine
    181–3, 191
molybdenum 180
monosodium glutamate (MSG) (E621)
    89, 96
mood 6
  and anti-nutrients 78, 85
  assessing your child's 106
  and blood sugar balance 136–7
  enhancement 135–45
  and food allergies 97
  and neurotransmitters 139–41
  and vitamins 72
motivation 139, 140
MSM (sulphur) 180
muesli 240
multivitamins and minerals 67–8, 107
  and aggressive behaviour 196
  chewable 113, 252
  choosing 251–2
  and heavy metals 84
  and IQ 2, 108–11, 113, 116
  and mood 145
  and reading/writing skills 127
mutagens 88
myelin sheaths 43–4, **43**, **44**, 55

National Autistic Society 171
Needleman, Herbert 82
nervous system, enteric 223
net protein usability (NPU) 63
neuronal connections 14–16, **15**
neurons 14, **15**, **43**
neurotransmitters 16–17, **17**, 57, 103, 108
  and epilepsy 190
  and mood 139–41
  protein and 60, 61–3
  supplementing for balance 141–4, *142*
  types of 61–2
night vision 153
nitrosamines 89
noradrenalin 62, 139, 140, 142–4, 165,
    166
nursery food 245
nutritional supplements 249–53, *250–1*
nuts 97, 121
Nystatin 181, 184

oat cakes 121
oats 97
obesity 220
Oliver, Jamie 2, 248
Omega-3 essential fats 40
  action in the body 42–4

Omega-3 essential fats – *contd*
  for ADHD 156, 158–60
  and aggressive behaviour 195–6
  and breastfeeding 219–20
  for epilepsy 189
  for the eyes 132–3
  fat family of 47, **47**
  and intelligence 41–2, 110, 113–16
  for mood 138–9, 144, 145
  recommended intake 46, **46**, 48
  sources 47–9, 50–2, 81, *81–2*, 160, 234
  supplementation 4, 51–2, 113–15, *115*, 253
Omega-6 essential fats 40, 49–52
  action in the body 42–4
  for epilepsy 189
  fat family of 49, **49**
  and intelligence 41–2
  recommended intake 46, **46**
  sources 49–52, 50–2
  supplementation 4, 51–2
organic produce 48, 91–2, 223–4, 236
organophosphates 134
Osmond, Humphry 166–7
Owens, Judith 210–11

pancreas 22
Papalos, Demitri 197
parabens 89
Pauling, Linus 109
pectin 83
peptides, exorphins 176–7, 178, 180, 207
periwinkle 190
pesticides 91, 134
Pfeiffer, Carl 187
phenylalanine 16, 142, 144, 145
phenytoin 186
phospholipids 18, 44, 55–9
  checking your child's levels of 55–6
  and epilepsy 189–91
  phosphatidyl choline 56–7, 59, 122–3, 125–6, 189, 253
  phosphatidyl serine 56, 57, 59, 123, 126
  sources 55, 57–9
  supplementation 58, 253
physical exercise 139, 140, 214, 215
physical intelligence (PQ) 41, 104
ponceau 4R, cochineal red A (E124) 89
porridge 240
potassium benzoate (E212) *see* calcium benzoate (E213)
potassium nitrate (E249) 89
pregnancy 12–14, 219
  essential fat intake during 41–2, 48
pregnancy – *contd*
  phospholipid intake during 56
  vitamin/mineral intake during 69, 73, 133, *133*
preservatives 86, 88–90, 235
prison diets 137–8
probiotics 177, 227
propyl p-hydroxy-benzoate, propyl-paraben, paraben (E216) 89
protein 60–6, 103
  checking your child's levels of 61
  food combining 32–3, 38, 158
  net protein usability 63
  portions 241
  problems digesting 177
  requirements *63*, 64–5
  sources 64, *64–5*, 65–6
  supplementation 60–1, 65–6
psychosis 4
pulses 242–3
pumpkin seed butter 240–1
pumpkin seeds 50, 51
Puri, Basant 138–9
pyroglutamate 123, 124–5, 126, 253
pyroluria 173, 177, 191

raw foods 239
reading ability
  assessing your child's 105–6
  foods for 42, 127–34
receptors 16, **17**
recommended daily allowance (RDA) 111–12
reduced-fat products 236–7
restaurants 232
reward deficiency syndrome 168–9
rhinitis 87–91
rhodopsin 134
Richardson, Alex 4, 42, 152
rickets 220
Rimland, Bernard 5, 123, 166–7, 173, 182
Ritalin 62, 123, 164–9, 182–3
Roberts, Gwillym 2, 67, 109
Rogers, Peter 37
Rooibosch tea 36
rye 97

saccharin (E954) 90
salicylates 94, 161–2, 179
salmon 48
SAMe (s-adenosyl methionine) 143, 189
schizophrenia 76
Schoenthaler, Stephen 109, 163, 196

school meals 2, 245–8
school vending machines 118
seed foods 64
seed oils 51–2, 54
seeds 51, 54, *64*, 121
    see also specific seeds
selenium 39, 75
    and aggressive behaviour 196
    and epilepsy 188
    and heavy metals 79, 80, 84
    supplementation 79
serotonin 16, 62, 72
    and eating disorders 205–7
    and mood 138–44
    and sleep 213
Seroxat 62–3
sesame seeds 50, 51
shellfish 97
shopping lists 235
sleep apnoea 212–13
sleep problems 78, 85, 209–15
smoking 73, 77, 80
snacks
    Glycemic Load of **29–30**
    healthy 121, 125, 231, 235–6, 242,
        246–7
    ideas for 242
    sugary 118
Snowden, Wendy 110
sodium metabisulphite (E223) 90
sodium sulphite (E221) 90
soya 97, 180
speech and language delay 21, 39
spina bifida 73
sprouts 243
stannous chloride (E512) 90
starflower/borage oil 49, 52
steam-frying 243
steaming 239
Stordy, Jacqueline 152–3
Strattera 165
stress 139–41
sugar
    family **26**
    fruit content 25, 31–2
    hidden 21, 120, 234
sugar, refined (anti-nutrient) 18, 22, 118
    and ADHD 156–7
    lack of nutrients 24–5
    substitutes for 32
    weaning kids off 31–2, 38
sulphation 180
sulphite oxidase 180
sulphur dioxide (E220) 90

sunflower seeds 50, 51
sunset yellow FCF, orange/yellow S
    (E110) 90
supermarkets 233–7
synapses **15**, 16

tannins 36
tantrums 235
tartrazine (E102) 86, 91
taurine 190
tea 36
television 210–11, 215
theobromine 35, 36
theophylline 36
thimerosal 182–3
This Morning (TV programme) 4, 128–9
toast 240–1
Tonight with Trevor McDonald (TV
    programme) 4
tri-methyl-glycine (TMG) 143, 145,
    189
tryptamines 62
tryptophan 16, 60, 213
    and appetite 203, 205–7
    and mood 136, 141–2
    natural sources of 141–2
5-hydroxy-tryptophan (5-HTP) 142–3,
    144, 145, 206, 213, 215
tummy ache 93–4
tuna 48, 114
tyrosine 60–1, 136, 142–3, 144, 145

unhappiness 136–40
urticaria 87–91

valine 205
vegetables
    getting kids to eat 238–9
    organic 91–2
    protein content of *65*
vegetarians
    and anorexia nervosa 205
    omega-3 intake 48
    phospholipid intake 58
    protein sources for 64, 66
vinpocetine 190
vitamin A (retinol) *133*
    and autism 174–5
    cautions regarding 133–4
    for the eyes 132–3
vitamin B1 (thiamine) *69*, 70, 71–2
    for epilepsy 188
    and IQ 112
    and memory 122

vitamin B3 (niacin) *69*, 70, 72
  and ADHD 159
  and mood 137
vitamin B5 (pantothenic acid) *69*, 70, 72,
  122
vitamin B6 70, *70*, 72–3
  and ADHD 159, 166, 167
  and autism 173, 176
  and eating disorders 206
  and epilepsy 186–7
  and IQ 112
  and mood 137
  for sleep problems 213
  and zinc 188
vitamin B12 70, *70*, 72–3
  and IQ 112
  and memory 122
  and mood 137
vitamin B complex *69–70*, 70–3, 107
  and epilepsy 186–7
  and homocysteine levels 14, 71
  and mood 137, 144
  and school grades 14
  sources *69–70*, 70
vitamin C *70*, 74, 75
  and ADHD 159, 166
  and autism 173
  and dyslexia/dyspraxia 153
  and heavy metals 79, 84
  and IQ 108
  and memory 122
  supplementation 252
vitamin D 188, 220
vitamin E 74, 75, 188, 220
vitamins 18, 67–75, 77
  checking your child's intake of 68
  IQ boosting 67–8, 69, 108–11,
    112–13, 113
  key **69–70**
  and mood 136, 137, 144
  sources 25
  supplementation 249–53, *250*
  toxicity of 251–2

vitamins – *contd*
  see also multivitamins and minerals;
    specific vitamins
Volkow, Nora 164

Wakefield, Andrew 177, 181–2
Ward, Neil 86, 162–3
weaning 219, 221–2, 224–5, 227
weaning diaries 222
wheat
  allergies to 96–7, 99, 175, 178–80, 183
  and binge eating 207
wholefoods 24–5, 37–8, 236, 239
wholegrains 38
Willatts, Peter 41
World Health Organization (WHO) 48
Wozniak, Janet 197
writing skills
  assessing your child's 105–6
  foods for 127–34, **129–30**
Wurtman, Richard 57

xylitol 32

yeast-containing foods 96–7
yoghurt 226
young offenders 4, 137–8, 157, 163, 194,
  196
Yudkin, John 109

zinc 14, *70*, 76–7, 138
  and ADHD 159, 162, 163, 166
  and aggressive behaviour 196
  and autism 176–7
  deficiency 39, 107, 202–3
  and dyslexia/dyspraxia 153
  and eating disorders 76, 202–5, 206
  effect of food additives on 86
  and epilepsy 188
  and heavy metals 79, 80, 81, 84
  and IQ 111–12
  and mood 137
  supplementation 79, 252